CONTENTS

Introduction

This Air fryer Oven Cookbook contains easy, delicious, and healthy recipes that can be prepared within few minutes. It is highly recommended for people with busy schedules and also for those on the Weight Watchers Program.

Even if you have never tried the Air Fryer Oven before, it promises you one thing, after having this cookbook, you will be kicking yourself for having not discovered this sooner.

It will inspire you to clean up your kitchen from all the useless appliances that clutter your countertop and start putting the Air Fryer Oven to good use. The air fryer oven will give you lots of joy, time, and, most importantly, tasty dishes. Feel free to adjust and alter these recipes, or simply use them as a springboard of inspiration for your own creations!

The Air Fryer Oven is definitely a change in lifestyle that will make things much easier for you and your family. You'll discover increased energy, decreased hunger, a boosted metabolism, and of course, a LOT of free time! You will know that it is not just a simple kitchen appliance. Still, it's truly a kitchen-miracle that will bring relief and satisfaction with its user-friendly functions, time plus energy-effective heating method, and multiple cooking options. This cookbook will share as many different recipes to provide an extensive guideline to all the frequent oven users. With the latest air fryer oven functions, you can air fry, dehydrate, broil, toast, roast, and bake all kinds of the dishes. Please give it a full read and find out tons of new ways to add more colors and flavors to your dinner table using the Air fryer Oven.

Why Use an Air Fryer Oven?

First and foremost, the air fryer oven became popular for its numerous health benefits. The convenience and ease of using an air fryer oven give an effortless choice for people that wants a healthy and delicious meal in a matter of time. For those who are hesitant on the air fryer oven potential and favor the conventional cooking way, perhaps the following benefits are enough to assure them to make the switch to efficient cooking:

- Great for cooking solidified foods without oil and extraordinary or pre-heating foods.
- Because of littler bins, the food cooked speedier when contrasted with ovens, and no pre-heating is fundamental.
- The kind of food is brilliant because the heat gives a pleasantly fresh and does not burn.
- Perfect for two individuals or littler segments. There's such a significant number of greater models out there to cook bigger parts for multiple individuals. The potential outcomes are inestimable.

- It's a healthier method of cooking fried or crispy foods. In general, you can utilize substantially less oil to accomplish crunchy and crispy finished foods.
- There's tidy little up and less splattering of oil while cooking. Everything gets contained pleasantly inside the air fryer while cooking.
- Food cooks fresh due to the littler cooking zone, and the heating component is nearer to the food.
- There's no need to warm up your home in summer when you're longing for something warm, roasted, or pan-fried.

Cleaning and Maintenance

Remember to clean your air fryer oven and accessories according to the instructions and safety precautions after each cooking adventure. Like every appliance, maintenance is needed to get what you would like in the device. Any tool employed for preparing food must be stored spotlessly clean. Don't let dirt develop and clean the environment fryer frequently, so you get great results when you make use of the air fryer oven. You have to make sure you remember it, "keep clean and maintain it" for best results efficiently because taken care of the appliance will always last longer. We provide you with some cleaning tips; however, it is not difficult. The outdoors and inside parts could be cleaned relatively easily and ought to be done frequently. Within the situation from the heating coil, get it done a couple of occasions annually only.

With so many recipes and a comprehensive guideline about the air fryer oven, you will know how to put to its best use and enjoy a range of flavorsome crispy meals in no time. This ten in one multipurpose kitchen miracle has brought much-wanted peace and comfort to the homemakers' lives who can now cook a healthy and delicious meal for their family in no time. This cookbook's different segment provides a step-by-step direction to cook various meals ranging from breakfast, poultry, meat, vegetables, snacks, and much more. Get this latest hit Air Fryer Oven Cookbook and bring convenience to your kitchen floor now. If you had an air fryer oven and you don't know what to cook in it, now you do – with all the recipes at its best!

What are you still waiting for? Start cooking in your air fryer oven and enjoy all the foods you thought were not healthy!

Chapter 1. How to Use Kalorik Digital Maxx Air Fryer Oven?

Having a Kalorik Air Fryer Oven is already a pretty big reason to bring this beauty home. But there are actual cooking advantages that this efficient Kalorik Air Fryer Oven offers you.

Modern Design

The design of the Maxx Air Fryer oven is something that makes it stand out among the rest of the air fryer ovens in the market. Its size and shape make a complete balance; you can manage cooking space and your countertop space simultaneously. Since this oven can replace multiple food appliances due to various its cooking functions, it can be easily placed anywhere in the kitchen.

Multi-functional

This one appliance can replace most of the cooking appliances in your kitchen as it provides several cooking functions in one place. This Air Fryer oven can be used to bake food, toast, grill, roast, braise, rotisserie, broil, and dehydrate all sorts of food items. Its cooking function's versatility increases when you count the temperature and timer settings, which can also be adjusted manually to cook according to your own preferences. Several attachments come with the oven, and they all help to cook on a specific cooking mode. There are 21 presets given in the appliance, which allows you to cook various meals.

Modern French Door System

One of the most exciting features of this Air fryer oven is its French door system, which opens from the center with a single-hand opening. Due to this feature, there is no dripping and scalding on its door during each cooking session. The French door system also makes it easy to check the food or to handle it during cooking. Moreover, it provides you complete space to insert a large tray or pan inside the Air Fryer oven.

Family Size

The 26-quart Maxx Air fryer oven is known for its large size and capacity, suitable for cooking all portion sizes. If you have a big or a small family, this Air fryer oven can serve the needs of all. Now baking a turkey and roasting a whole chicken or a duck is not a problem, as you can not only adjust them all in this Air Fryer oven, but you can also add side ingredients along with them.

Simple and Smart Control Panel

Another useful feature of this Air Fryer oven is its easy and simple control panel, which is ultimately user friendly. There are two main buttons to choose between the Air Fryer options or baking options. And the control dial is used to select the mode of cooking in each option.

How to Use Kalorik Digital Maxx Air Fryer Oven?

Here are a few simple steps to use your Kalorik Digital Maxx Air Fryer Oven:

Getting Started

At first, place the appliance at an appropriate place in the kitchen. The back and top of the oven should be kept open for ventilation. Check all its accessories and then plug it in. The lights of the display screen will light up.

If you are using the oven for the first time, make sure to wash all the accessories with water or soap water and allow them to dry, and keep them at a place where they are safe from the dirt and grease.

Setting Up the oven

The crumb tray is placed at the inside bottom of the oven, and it is essential to use this tray to protect the oven's floor. So always fix the crumb tray in the lowermost portion of the oven. You can now select the accessories according to the recipe and the type of food. The air fryer basket is used to Air Fry various food items, so use this basket to keep the food inside the oven. The baking pan and tray can be used for a variety of purpose:

- To bake food
- To roast items
- To Broil
- To toast

The Rotisserie rod and handle are provided to cook on the chicken, duck, etc. on the rotisserie. The chicken or duck is heated correctly from each side as the rod rotates and gets an equal brown color on all sides.

The dehydrator tray is used for dehydrating meat, fruits, and vegetables. And there is also a bacon tray that is used for cooking crispy bacon in the oven. You can use the accessories according to your needs. There is also an Air Rack, which you can use for Air frying and roasting or baking etc.

Cooking and Adjustment

Now that you have selected the desired accessories for cooking. Prepare your food and keep it ready for the oven. The oven quickly attains the required heat for cooking, so it is suggested not to preheat the oven and directly place the food inside and then select the cooking functions. You can change the settings according to the given recipe. Generally, it is best to select after your food is placed inside.

Once the food is set inside, close the French glass doors to seal the oven and then select any of the two options: AIR FRY or OVEN, then use the dial to select the required preset to adjust the time-temperature. When the appliance starts actual cooking, the timer starts ticking, and you will notice the magic happening inside the oven through its glass doors. If you want to flip or toss the food inside the oven, then simply press STOP to pause the cooking function and flip or toss the food. Close the doors again and resume cooking by pressing the START button. You can always use the LIGHT function to check your food's status and prevent it from burning, overcooking, or undercooking.

Once the operation is completed, the appliance will indicate a beep or a blink on the screen. It is wise to leave the food for 5-10 minutes in the oven and then dish out for safe and easy handling. When you are done cooking, remove the food from the oven along with all the accessories used.

Cleaning and Maintenance

No cooking appliance can work longer if it is not cleaned or maintained correctly, especially an Air Fryer oven like this oven needs all the care and attention to keep it suitable for cooking clean and hygienic food. Inside the oven, when food particles or dirty accessories are left without cleaning, it can cause bacterial growth, contaminating the food placed inside. So, here are few simple steps to clean the appliance after every cooking session.

First, unplug the appliance and remove all the trays or pans placed inside. Make sure to wear gloves or oven mittens while handling the hot trays. It is essential to clean the tray and pan while they are hot to prevent all the grease and food particles stuck on them from hardening.

Leave the cooking appliance with its door open and allow it to cool completely.

Use this time to wash all the accessories used in the cooking operation. You can either wash them by lightly rub them with soap water or wash them in the dishwasher. Avoid using hard material to scrub these accessories, as they could damage their outer surface.

Once the accessories are washed, leave them to dry completely.

Now that the oven is cooled from inside out, you can take a lightly damp cloth and wipe off all the grease and food particles from the inner walls of the Air Fryer oven.

Use another lightly wet cloth to wipe off the doors, door handle, the control panel dial, buttons, and the displace screen.

Never immerse the unit water and keep it away from liquids as well.

Chapter 2. Air Fryer Oven Tips & Tricks and Its Function Keys

Air fryer Ovens are designed to be super easy to use. Here's a little tip to get you started:

Choosing A Recipe

Choose a recipe that you can cook in your air fryer. Remember that most foods you cook in your microwave or oven, or on the stovetop, can be prepared in the air fryer - except for those recipes with a lot of fat or liquids. You can use my air fryer cookbook to help you find suitable recipes.

Preparing the Air Fryer

Read through the recipe to the end, so you know what accessories you need for cooking. Some recipes call for using the basket, rack, or rotisserie that comes with the air fryer. Other recipes use cake or muffin pans that you can insert into the air fryer. Just be sure these pans fit into the fryer and are safe to use.

Preparing the Ingredients

Gather the ingredients for the recipe and prep them according to the instructions. When prepped, put the ingredients into the air fryer or in the basket, rack, or pans within the air fryer. Use parchment baking paper or a light mist of oil spray to prevent food from sticking.

Never crowd food in the air fryer or over-fill. Food that is crowded in the air fryer won't cook evenly and can be raw and under-cooked. If you're preparing for a crowd, you may have to cook more than one batch.

Setting the Temperature and Time

Check the recipe for the correct temperature and time setting. You can set manually; you can use the digital setting for the temperature and time needed for the recipe. Most air fryers also have preset functions that make it easy to set according to each recipe.

Check Food During Cooking

Many air fryer oven recipes require you to check the food while cooking so that it cooks evenly and doesn't over-cook. You will need to shake, flip, or toss the food to distribute it. Or for some recipes, you'll need to turn the food about halfway through when cooking so that it cooks and crisps all the way thoroughly.

Cleaning the Air Fryer

Once the food is cooked, remove and unplug the air fryer. Let it cool completely before cleaning. Follow the directions that come with the air fryer oven for proper cleaning. Never scrub or use abrasive cleaners when cleaning the fryer or the fryer accessories.

Using the Basket or Rack

Some air fryers use a round basket where foods are cooked, while other models will have layered racks that fit into a square cooking space, much like a small oven. Most of the recipes given in this cookbook can be used for both baskets and racks.

Keep an Eye on Timing

You'll find that air fryers cook at different temperatures depending on what model you have. It is why it's essential to check on foods during the cooking process, so you don't over or undercook them. If you've cut back on quantities in some of the recipes, be sure to cut the cooking time down accordingly. Remember, hints are just recommendations to guide you as you use your air fryer.

Using Oil Sprays

Most of the recipes use an oil spray. But if you desire, you can use any brand you want. Or make your own by merely putting olive oil into a small spray bottle. Use a small amount of oil and spray over the basket and trays to prevent food from sticking. Some of the recipes require you to spray the food with oil directly.

Function Keys

The following are the functions keys of an Air Fryer Oven:

Play/Pause Button

This Play/Pause button allows you to pause during the middle of the cooking so you can shake the air fryer basket or flip the food to ensure it cooks evenly.

-/+ Button /Minus or Plus Button

This button is used to change the time or temperature.

Keep Warm

This function keeps your food warm for 30 minutes.

Food Presets

This button gives you the ability to cook food without second-guessing. The time and temperature are already set, so new users find this setting useful.

Roast or Broil

You can roast or broil with this setting. When using a conventional oven, you need to brown the meat before roasting. You can skip this step when cooking with an air fryer.

Dehydrate

This setting cooks and dries food at a low temperature for a few hours. With this option, you can create your beef jerky or dried fruit.

Chapter 3. Breakfast Recipes

1. Air Fryer Baked Eggs

Preparation time: 5 minutes
Cooking time: 7 minutes
Servings: 2

Ingredients:

2 large eggs
2 tablespoons half-and-half
2 teaspoons shredded Cheddar cheese
Salt
ground black pepper
Cooking spray

Directions:

Spritz 2 ramekins lightly with cooking spray. Crack an egg into each ramekin.
Top each egg with 1 tablespoon of half-and-half and 1 teaspoon of Cheddar cheese. Sprinkle with salt and black pepper. Stir the egg mixture with a fork until well combined.
Place the ramekins in the air fryer oven—Cook at 330ºF (166ºC) for 6 minutes.
Allow cooling for 5 minutes before removing and serving.

Nutrition:

Calories: 143
Carbs: 1g
Fat: 10g
Protein: 13g

2. Asparagus and Cheese Strata

Preparation time: 10 minutes
Cooking time: 17 minutes
Servings: 4

Ingredients:

6 asparagus spears, cut into 2-inch pieces
1 tablespoon water
2 slices whole-wheat bread, cut into ½-inch cubes
4 eggs
3 tablespoons whole milk
2 tablespoons chopped flat-leaf parsley
½ cup grated Havarti or Swiss cheese
Pinch salt
Freshly ground black pepper, to taste
Cooking spray

Directions:

Add the asparagus spears and 1 tablespoon of water in a baking pan.
Cook at 330ºF (166ºC) for 4 minutes in the air fryer oven.
Remove the asparagus from the pan and drain on paper towels.
Spritz the pan with cooking spray. Place the bread and asparagus in the pan.
Mix the eggs plus milk in a medium mixing bowl until creamy. Fold in the parsley, cheese, salt, and pepper and stir to combine. Pour this mixture into the baking pan.
Put the basket again to the air fryer oven—Bake for 13 minutes. When done, the eggs will be set, and the top will be lightly browned.
Let it cool for 5 minutes before slicing and serving.

Nutrition:

Calories: 240
Carbs: 16g
Fat: 11g
Protein: 19g

3. Bacon and Egg Bread Cups

Preparation time: 15 minutes
Cooking time: 10 minutes
Servings: 4

Ingredients:

4 (3-by-4-inch) crusty rolls
4 thin slices Gouda or Swiss cheese mini wedges
5 eggs
2 tablespoons heavy cream
3 strips precooked bacon, chopped
½ teaspoon dried thyme
Pinch salt
Freshly ground black pepper, to taste

Directions:

On a clean work surface, cut the tops off the rolls.
Using your fingers, remove the rolls' insides to make bread cups, leaving a ½-inch shell. Place a slice of cheese onto each roll bottom.
Whisk the eggs and heavy cream in a medium bowl until well combined. Fold in the bacon, thyme, salt, and pepper and stir well.
Scrape the egg mixture into the prepared bread cups.
Place the bread cups into the air fryer oven—Cook at 330ºF (166ºC) for 10 minutes.
When cooked, the eggs should be cooked to your preference.
Serve warm.

Nutrition:

Calories: 140
Carbs: 0g
Fat: 11g
Protein: 10g

4. Baked Avocado with Eggs

Preparation time: 5 minutes
Cooking time: 9 minutes
Servings: 2

Ingredients:

1 large avocado, halved and pitted
2 large eggs
2 tomato slices, divided
½ cup nonfat Cottage cheese, divided
½ teaspoon fresh cilantro, for garnish

Directions:

Line the sheet pan with the aluminum foil.
Slice a thin piece from the bottom of each avocado half, so they sit flat. Remove a small amount from each avocado half to make a bigger hole to hold the egg.
Arrange the avocado halves on the pan, hollow side up. Break 1 egg into each half. Then top with 1 tomato slice and ¼ cup of the Cottage cheese.
Cook in the air fryer at 425ºF (220ºC) for 9 minutes.
Garnish with the fresh cilantro and serve.

Nutrition:

Calories: 355
Carbs: 9g
Fat: 29g
Protein: 17g

5. Banana and Oat Bread Pudding

Preparation time: 10 minutes
Cooking time: 16 minutes
Servings: 4

Ingredients:

2 medium ripe bananas, mashed
½ cup low-fat milk
2 tablespoons maple syrup
2 tablespoons peanut butter
1 teaspoon vanilla extract
1 teaspoon ground cinnamon
2 slices whole-grain bread, cut into bite-sized cubes
¼ cup quick oats
Cooking spray

Directions:

Spritz a baking dish lightly with cooking spray.
Mix the bananas, milk, maple syrup, peanut butter, vanilla, and cinnamon in a large mixing bowl and stir until well incorporated.
Add the bread cubes to the banana mixture and stir until thoroughly coated. Fold in the oats and stir to combine.
Transfer the mixture to the baking dish. Wrap the baking dish in aluminum foil.
Slide the baking dish into the air fryer oven—Cook at 350ºF (180ºC) for 16 minutes.
After 10 minutes, remove the foil. Return and continue to cook another 6 minutes.
When done, the pudding should be set. Let the pudding cool for 5 minutes before serving.

Nutrition:

Calories: 132
Carbs: 21g
Fat: 4g
Protein: 3g

6. Blueberry Cake

Preparation time: 5 minutes
Cooking time: 10 minutes
Servings: 8

Ingredients:

1½ cups Bisquick
¼ cup granulated sugar
2 large eggs, beaten
¾ cup whole milk
1 teaspoon vanilla extract
½ teaspoon lemon zest
Cooking spray
2 cups blueberries

Directions:

Stir the Bisquick and sugar in a medium bowl. Stir the eggs, milk, vanilla, and lemon zest. Add the wet ingredients to the dry ingredients and stir until well combined.
Spritz the sheet pan with cooking spray and line with the parchment paper, pressing it into place.
Spray the parchment paper with cooking spray. Put the batter on the pan and spread it out evenly.
Sprinkle the blueberries evenly over the top.
Put into the air fryer oven. Cook at 375ºF (190ºC) for 10 minutes.
Let the cake rest for a minute before cutting into 16 squares. Serve immediately.

Nutrition:

Calories: 140
Carbs: 16g
Fat: 7g
Protein: 2g

7. Breakfast Cheese Sandwiches

Preparation time: 5 minutes
Cooking time: 8 minutes
Servings: 2

Ingredients:

1 teaspoon butter, softened
4 slices bread
4 slices smoked country ham
4 slices Cheddar cheese
4 thick slices tomato

Directions:

Spoon ½ teaspoon of butter onto one side of 2 slices of bread and spread it all over.
Assemble the sandwiches: Top each of 2 slices of unbuttered bread with 2 pieces of ham, 2 slices of cheese, and 2 slices of tomato. Place the remaining 2 slices of bread on top, butter-side up.
Lay the sandwiches in an air fryer basket, buttered side down.
Put the basket into the air fryer oven—Cook at 370ºF (188ºC) for 8 minutes.
Flip the sandwiches halfway through the cooking time.
Allow cooling for 5 minutes before slicing to serve.

Nutrition:

Calories: 385
Carbs: 29g
Fat: 20g
Protein: 23g

8. Breakfast Tater Tot Casserole

Preparation time: 5 minutes
Cooking time: 18 minutes
Servings: 4

Ingredients:

4 eggs
1 cup milk
Salt and pepper, to taste
12 ounces (340 g) ground chicken sausage
1 pound (454 g) frozen tater tots, thawed
¾ cup grated Cheddar cheese
Cooking spray

Directions:

Mix the eggs, including milk, in a medium bowl. Put salt plus pepper to taste and stir until mixed. Set aside.
Place a skillet over medium-high heat and spritz with cooking spray. Place the ground sausage in the skillet and break it into smaller pieces with a spatula or spoon. Cook for 3 to 4 minutes until the sausage browns, stirring occasionally. Remove from heat and set aside.
Coat a baking pan with cooking spray. Arrange the tater tots in the baking pan.

Cook in the air fryer oven at 400ºF (205ºC) for 14 minutes.

After 6 minutes, remove then stir the tater tots, add the egg mixture, and cooked sausage. Return and cook again.

Remove again, then scatter the cheese on top of the tater tots. Continue to cook another 2 minutes.

Let the batter cool for 5 minutes and serve warm.

Nutrition:

Calories: 217

Carbs: 9g

Fat: 14g

Protein: 13g

9. Canadian Bacon Muffin Sandwiches

Preparation time: 5 minutes

Cooking time: 8 minutes

Servings: 4

Ingredients:

4 English muffins, split

8 slices Canadian bacon

4 slices cheese

Cooking spray

Directions:

Make the sandwiches: Top each of 4 muffin halves with 2 pieces of Canadian bacon, 1 slice of cheese, and finish with the remaining muffin half.

Put the sandwiches in an air fryer basket and spritz the tops with cooking spray.

Cook at 370ºF (188ºC) for 8 minutes.

Flip the sandwiches halfway through the cooking time.

Divide the sandwiches among four plates and serve warm.

Nutrition:

Calories: 220

Carbs: 25g

Fat: 8g

Protein: 12g

10. Carrot Banana Muffin

Preparation time: 10 minutes

Cooking time: 20 minutes

Servings: 12

Ingredients:

1½ cups whole-wheat flour

1 cup grated carrot

1 cup mashed banana

½ cup bran

½ cup low-fat buttermilk

2 tablespoons agave nectar

2 teaspoons baking powder

1 teaspoon vanilla

1 teaspoon baking soda

½ teaspoon nutmeg

Pinch cloves

2 egg whites

Directions:

Line your muffin pan using 12 paper liners.

In a large bowl, stir all the fixing. Mix well, but do not overbeat.

Scoop the mixture into the muffin cups.

Put the pan into the air fryer oven—Cook at 400ºF (205ºC) for 20 minutes.

Serve warm or at room temperature.

Nutrition:

Calories: 235

Carbs: 27g

Fat: 2g

Protein: 5g

11. Cheesy Artichoke-Mushroom Frittata

Preparation time: 10 minutes

Cooking time: 15 minutes

Servings: 6

Ingredients:

8 eggs

½ teaspoon kosher salt

¼ cup whole milk

¾ cup shredded Mozzarella cheese, divided

2 tablespoons unsalted butter, melted

1 cup coarsely chopped artichoke hearts

¼ cup chopped onion

½ cup mushrooms

¼ cup grated Parmesan cheese

¼ teaspoon freshly ground black pepper

Directions:

Mix the eggs and salt in a medium bowl, rest it for a minute or two, and then pour in the milk and whisk again. Stir in ½ cup of the Mozzarella cheese.

Grease a sheet pan with the butter. Stir in the artichoke hearts and onion and toss to coat with the butter.

Put into the air fryer oven. Cook at 375ºF (190ºC) for 12 minutes.

After 5 minutes, remove the pan. Spread the mushrooms over the vegetables. Pour the egg mixture on top. Stir gently just to distribute the vegetables evenly.

Return and continue cooking for 10 minutes, or until the edges are set. The center will still be liquid.

After 1 minute, remove the pan and sprinkle the remaining ¼ cup of the Mozzarella and Parmesan cheese over the frittata. Return it and continue to cook again.

Sprinkle the black pepper on top and serve.

Nutrition:

Calories: 196

Carbs: 7g

Fat: 15g

Protein: 10g

12. Cheesy Breakfast Casserole

Preparation time: 10 minutes

Cooking time: 16 minutes

Servings: 4

Ingredients:

6 slices bacon

6 eggs

Salt and pepper, to taste

Cooking spray

½ cup chopped green bell pepper

½ cup chopped onion

¾ cup shredded Cheddar cheese

Directions:

Put the bacon in a skillet over medium-high heat and cook each side for about 4 minutes until evenly crisp.

Remove from the heat to a paper towel-lined plate to drain. Crumble it into small pieces and set aside.
Whisk the eggs with the salt and pepper in a medium bowl.
Spritz a baking pan with cooking spray.
Place the whisked eggs, crumbled bacon, green bell pepper, and onion in the prepared pan.
Put the pan into the air fryer oven—Cook at 400ºF (205ºC) for 8 minutes.
After 6 minutes, remove and scatter the Cheddar cheese all over. Return, then continue to cook within 2 minutes.
Let it sit for 5 minutes and serve on plates.

Nutrition:

Calories: 329
Carbs: 9g
Fat: 8g
Protein: 21g

13. Cheesy Hash Brown Casserole

Preparation time: 15 minutes
Cooking time: 30 minutes
Servings: 4

Ingredients:

3½ cups frozen hash browns, thawed
1 teaspoon salt
1 teaspoon freshly ground black pepper
3 tablespoons butter, melted
1 (10.5-ounce / 298-g) can cream of chicken soup
½ cup sour cream
1 cup minced onion
½ cup shredded sharp Cheddar cheese
Cooking spray

Directions:

Season the hash browns in a large bowl with salt and black pepper.
Add the melted butter, cream of chicken soup, and sour cream and stir until well incorporated. Mix in the minced onion and cheese well.
Spray a baking pan with cooking spray. Spread the hash brown batter into the baking pan.
Cook at 325ºF (163ºC) for 30 minutes. When cooked, the hash brown mixture will be browned.
Cool for 5 minutes before serving.

Nutrition:

Calories: 210
Carbs: 16g
Fat: 14g
Protein: 6g

14. Cheesy Hash Brown Cups

Preparation time: 10 minutes
Cooking time: 9 minutes
Servings: 6

Ingredients:

4 eggs, beaten
2¼ cups frozen hash browns, thawed
1 cup diced ham
½ cup shredded Cheddar cheese
½ teaspoon Cajun seasoning
Cooking spray

Directions:

Lightly spritz a 12-cup muffin tin with cooking spray.
Combine the beaten eggs, hash browns, diced ham, cheese, and Cajun seasoning in a medium bowl and stir until well blended.
Spoon a heaping 1½ tablespoons of egg mixture into each muffin cup.
Place the muffin tin into the air fryer oven—Cook at 350ºF (180ºC) for 9 minutes.
Cool-down for 5 to 10 minutes on a wire rack and serve warm.

Nutrition:

Calories: 120
Carbs: 5g
Fat: 8g
Protein: 6g

15. Chocolate Banana Bread

Preparation time: 10 minutes
Cooking time: 30 minutes
Servings: 4

Ingredients:

¼ cup of cocoa powder
6 tablespoons plus 2 teaspoons all-purpose flour, divided
½ teaspoon kosher salt
¼ teaspoon baking soda
1½ ripe bananas
1 large egg, whisked
¼ cup of vegetable oil
½ cup of sugar
3 tablespoons buttermilk or plain yogurt (not Greek)
½ teaspoon vanilla extract
6 tablespoons chopped white chocolate
6 tablespoons chopped walnuts

Directions:

Mix the cocoa powder, 6 tablespoons of the flour, salt, and baking soda in a medium bowl.
Mash the bananas with a fork in another medium bowl until smooth. Fold in the egg, oil, sugar, buttermilk, vanilla, and whisk until thoroughly combined. Then put the wet batter to the dry batter and stir until well incorporated.
Combine the white chocolate, walnuts, and the remaining 2 tablespoons of flour in a third bowl and toss to coat. Put this to the batter and stir until well incorporated. Pour the batter into a baking pan and smooth the top with a spatula.
Cook at 310ºF (154ºC) for 30 minutes in the air fryer oven.
When done, a toothpick inserted into the center of the bread should come out clean.
Cool-down on a wire rack for 10 minutes before serving.

Nutrition:

Calories: 116
Carbs: 16g
Fat: 6g
Protein: 2g

16. Cinnamon Buns

Preparation time: 15 minutes
Cooking time: 10 minutes
Servings: 3

Ingredients:

8 oz. container crescent rolls, refrigerated

1 tbsp. ground cinnamon
2 oz. raisins
1/3 cup butter
2 tbsp. sugar, granulated
1/3 cup pecans, chopped
cooking spray (olive oil)
maple syrup – 2 tbsp.
1/3 cup brown sugar

Directions:

In a saucepan, dissolve the butter completely.
Transfer to a dish and blend the maple syrup and brown sugar.
Layer one 8-inch pan with the olive oil spray.
Distribute the sugar into the pan and empty the raisins and pecans inside, stirring to incorporate.
In a glass dish, whisk the sugar and ground cinnamon.
Open the can of crescent rolls and place on a cutting board.
Slice the entire log of dough into eight individual pieces.
Cover the top and bottom of the dough pieces in cinnamon and sugar, and transfer the pan to the air fryer.
Adjust the settings to air crisp at 345° F for 5 minutes.
Turn over the individual buns and steam for another 5 minutes.
Take the pan out and move the buns to a serving plate.
Drizzle the remaining sugar liquid on the buns and serve immediately.

Nutrition:

Calories: 190
Carbs: 33g
Fat: 4g
Protein: 6g

17. Egg and Cheese Veggie Cups

Preparation time: 15 minutes
Cooking time: 14 minutes
Servings: 4

Ingredients:

cooking spray (olive oil)
large eggs - 4
1/4 tsp. salt
2 oz. half & half
cheddar cheese – 8oz, shredded
3 tsp. chopped cilantro
1/8 tsp. pepper

Directions:

Set the air fryer to the temperature of 300° F to heat.
Liberally spray 4 glass or ceramic ramekin dishes.
In a glass dish, blend the half & half, salt, cilantro, eggs, pepper, and 4 oz. of the shredded cheese until combined.
Evenly distribute the mixture to the greased dishes.
Move the dishes to the basket in the air fryer for 12 minutes.
Once the time has passed, sprinkle the remaining 4 oz. of shredded cheese on top of each dish.
Adjust the temperature to 400° F and broil for an additional 2 minutes.
Serve immediately and enjoy!

Nutrition:

Calories: 34
Carbs: 0g
Fat: 1g
Protein: 5g

18. Egg in a Hole

Preparation time: 15 minutes
Cooking time: 10 minutes
Servings: 1

Ingredients:

Salt – ¼ tsp.
1 slice toast
1 large egg
1/8 tsp. pepper
cooking spray (olive oil)

Directions:

Liberally spray the pan inside the air fryer with cooking spray.
Remove the middle of the slice of bread with a small cookie cutter and move to the pan.
Break the egg and put it into the middle of the slice of bread.
Set the air fryer to heat at 330°F and cook for 6 minutes.
Use a metal spatula to turn the bread over and steam for an additional 4 minutes.
Serve hot and enjoy.

Nutrition:

Calories: 172
Carbs: 16g
Fat: 8g
Protein: 8g

19. French Toast Sticks

Preparation time: 15 minutes
Cooking time: 8 minutes
Servings: 3

Ingredients:

1 tbsp. ground cinnamon
4 tbsp. butter
1 cup milk
5 large eggs
1/4 cup sugar, confectioner
12 slices Texas toast
1 tsp. vanilla extract

Directions:

In a hot saucepan, liquefy the butter completely.
Meanwhile, cut the bread into 3 separate pieces.
Using a glass dish, blend the vanilla extract, melted butter, milk, and eggs thoroughly.
In an additional glass dish, combine the sugar and ground cinnamon.
Dunk each slice of bread into the wet mixture and cover with the sugar mixture completely.
Transfer to a dish and blend the maple syrup and brown sugar.
Move to the air fryer basket and fry for approximately 8 minutes while setting at 350°F.
Remove the sticks from the air fryer and wait for approximately 5 minutes before serving.

Nutrition:

Calories: 220
Carbs: 36g
Fat: 6g
Protein: 5g

20. Ham and Cheese Omelet

Preparation time: 15 minutes
Cooking time: 10 minutes
Servings: 4
Ingredients:
Salt - 1/4 tsp.
Milk – 2 oz.
cheddar cheese - 1/4 cup shredded
6 tsp. ham, diced
1/3 tsp. thyme seasoning
2 tbsp. bell pepper, diced
6 tsp. mushrooms
2 large eggs
1/3 tsp. oregano seasoning
2 tbsp. onions, diced
1/3 tsp. paprika seasoning
cooking spray (olive oil)
Directions:
Cover a 3x6-inch pan with olive oil spray.
Whisk the milk, salt, and eggs until blended in a glass dish.
Combine the diced ham, bell pepper, mushrooms, and onions and stir until merged.
Transfer to the greased pan and move to the air fryer basket.
Adjust the air fryer to 350°F and heat for approximately 5 minutes.
In a glass dish, combine the thyme, oregano, and paprika seasons.
Open the lid and sprinkle the seasonings evenly over the top. Then dust with the shredded cheese.
Steam for an additional 5 minutes. Use a rubber scraper to place between the omelet and the pan to lift. Move to a serving plate and serve while hot.
Nutrition:
Calories: 200
Carbs: 4g
Fat: 14g
Protein: 13g

21. Hard-Boiled Eggs

Preparation time: 15 minutes
Cooking time: 16 minutes
Servings: 6
Ingredients:
6 large eggs, cold
4 cups of ice water
Directions:
Adjust the air fryer to 250°F and insert the wire accessory into the basket.
Place the refrigerated eggs into the wire rack and heat for 16 minutes.
Remove the eggs to a dish of ice water.
Once cooled, peel the eggs and serve immediately.
Nutrition:
Calories: 58
Carbs: 0g
Fat: 0g
Protein: 6g

22. Home Fries

Preparation time: 15 minutes
Cooking time: 25 minutes
Servings: 3
Ingredients:
1 tsp. salt
3 russet potatoes, cubed
1 tsp. chili powder
3 tbsp paprika seasoning
2 tbsp olive oil
1/2 tsp pepper
3 tbsp garlic powder
Directions:
Adjust the air fryer temperature to 400°F to heat.
Prepare the potatoes by scrubbing and chopping into cubes.
Using a glass dish, combine the cubed potatoes with paprika, olive oil, chili powder, and garlic powder until integrated.
In a single layer, assemble the potatoes in the air fryer basket—Fry for approximately 25 minutes.
Open the lid about every 10 minutes to toss the potatoes for it to be cooked thoroughly.
Remove from the basket, distribute to a serving dish, then serve immediately.
Nutrition:
Calories: 113
Carbs: 23g
Fat: 1g
Protein: 2g

23. Loaded Hash Browns

Preparation time: 15 minutes
Cooking time: 20 minutes
Servings: 4
Ingredients:
2 garlic cloves, chopped
3 russet potatoes
2 oz. onions, chopped
1/4 cup red peppers, chopped
2 tsp. olive oil
1/4 tsp. salt
2 oz. cup green peppers, chopped
1 tsp. paprika seasoning
6 cups cold water
1/8 tsp. pepper
Directions:
Scrub the potatoes and remove the skins with a knife or vegetable peeler.
Use a cheese grater to shred the potatoes entirely with the largest holes available. Transfer the potatoes to a glass dish.
Empty the cold water into the dish and saturate for approximately 20 minutes.
Empty the potatoes and remove the moisture thoroughly.
Set the air fryer to heat at 400°F.
In an additional glass dish, blend the potatoes, olive oil, salt, garlic powder, paprika powder, and pepper until completely covered.
Put the potatoes to the air fryer basket and steam for 10 minutes.
Open the lid and combine the onion, garlic, and peppers to the basket. Toss ingredients to incorporate.
Heat for an additional 10 minutes and take out of the basket.

Wait for approximately 5 minutes before serving.
Nutrition:
Calories: 307
Carbs: 29g
Fat: 11g
Protein: 23g

24. Maple-Glazed Bacon

Preparation time: 15 minutes
Cooking time: 8 minutes
Servings: 5
Ingredients:
3 tbsp brown sugar
2 tbsp water
8 slices bacon
2 tbsp maple syrup
Directions:
Adjust the air fryer to heat at 400°F. Remove the basket and cover the base with baking paper.
Empty the water into the base of the fryer while preheating.
In a glass dish, whisk the 2 tbsp of maple syrup and the 3 tbsp brown sugar.
Place the wire rack into the basket and arrange the bacon into a single layer.
Spread the sugar glaze on the bacon until completely covered.
Put the basket into the air fryer and steam for 8 minutes.
Move the bacon from the basket and wait about 5 minutes before serving hot.
Nutrition:
Calories: 230
Carbs: 1g
Fat: 22g
Protein: 7g

25. Sausage, Egg, and Cheese Biscuits

Preparation time: 15 minutes
Cooking time: 16 minutes
Servings: 6
Ingredients:
pepper - 1/8 tsp.
10.2 oz. can biscuits, flaky
1/8 tsp. salt
1 1/2 tsp. vegetable oil
2oz. sharp cheddar cheese, cubed in 10 pieces
1 1/2 large eggs
1/8 lb. sausage, ground
1 1/2 tsp. water
cooking spray (olive oil)
Directions:
Create an 8-inch circle of baking lining and set on the base of the air fryer's basket. Cover with cooking spray. Put a separate piece of baking lining to the side.
Using a hot skillet, empty the oil and brown the sausage for approximately 4 minutes while breaking into small pieces with a wooden spatula.
Whip 2 of the eggs in a dish and blend with pepper and salt.
Remove the browned meat to a separate glass dish.
Adjust the temperature to medium. Empty the egg mixture and heat for about 60 seconds, then combine with the cooked sausage dish and mix thoroughly.
In the meantime, section the biscuit pastry into 5 pieces and transfer to the baking lining sheet.
Compress each into a thin circle and spoon a generous tablespoon of the meat and eggs into the middle.
Set a cube of cheese on the filling and enclose completely by pinching the sides of the pastry.
In a glass dish, combine the water and remaining egg until smooth.
Put the egg wash to each of the biscuits, covering entirely.
Transfer to the basket with the pinched sides on the baking lining.
Adjust the temperature to 325°F and heat for 10 minutes.
Flip the biscuits carefully and continue steaming for 6 minutes more.
Remove the biscuits to a plate and enjoy!
Nutrition:
Calories: 170
Carbs: 14g
Fat: 10g
Protein: 6g

26. Sausage Patties

Preparation time: 15 minutes
Cooking time: 20 minutes
Servings: 6
Ingredients:
1/2 tsp onion powder
11 oz. of sausage, ground, and cold
1/2 tsp red chili flakes
1/4 tsp thyme seasoning
1/8 tsp salt
1/4 tsp paprika seasoning
1 1/2 tsp garlic, minced
1 tsp brown sugar
1/4 tsp cayenne pepper
1 tsp Tabasco sauce
1/8 tsp Pepper
Directions:
Cover a baking tray with baking lining and place it into the air fryer basket.
Mix by hand the cold ground sausage with all the listed seasonings, Tabasco sauce, and brown sugar.
Divide the meat into 6 sections and create individual patties.
Move the patties to the basket in a single layer and adjust the air fryer to heat at 370° F.
Heat for 10 minutes and turn the patties to the other side.
Continue to "broil" for 10 additional minutes.
Remove from basket to a serving platter and enjoy.
Nutrition:
Calories: 190
Carbs: 2g
Fat: 14g
Protein: 12g

27. Savory Bagel Bites

Preparation time: 15 minutes

Cooking time: 9 minutes
Servings: 4
Ingredients:
1 cup self-rising flour
8 oz. Greek yogurt
1/2 cup cream cheese, whipped
cooking spray (olive oil)
Directions:
In a food blender, beat the yogurt and flour until it thickens into a dough for about 2 minutes.
Cover the base of the pan with cooking spray.
Create equal sized balls of the dough and move to the greased pan.
Shut the air fryer top and adjust the temperature to 325°F for about 5 minutes.
Turn the balls over and reset at the same temperature on the air crisp setting for 4 minutes.
Remove the balls from the basket and let it cool for approximately 10 minutes.
Poke a little hole into the sides of the bagels.
Pack the whipped cream cheese inside the holes using a pastry bag and serve immediately.
Nutrition:
Calories: 190
Carbs: 31g
Fat: 5g
Protein: 7g

28. Stuffed Baked Avocado

Preparation time: 15 minutes
Cooking time: 14 minutes
Servings: 2
Ingredients:
Two eggs, preferably large
Salt - 1/4 tsp.
1 avocado, large
3 tsp parsley seasoning
2 oz cheddar, shredded
1/8 tsp Pepper
Directions:
Set the air fryer to the temperature of 400°F.
Pit the avocado by slicing in half and break the eggs into the hollow of the avocado.
Sprinkle the pepper, parsley, and salt on top of the whole of the avocados.
Move the avocado halves into the basket and heat for approximately 14 minutes.
Remove, then transfer to a serving plate and dust with the shredded cheese before serving.
Nutrition:
Calories: 316
Carbs: 10g
Fat: 26g
Protein: 14g

29. Sweet Potato Toast

Preparation time: 15 minutes
Cooking time: 30 minutes
Servings: 4
Ingredients:
1/4 tsp Salt
1/8 tsp paprika seasoning
4 tsp avocado oil
1/8 tsp garlic powder
1 sweet potato
1/8 tsp onion powder
1/4 tsp pepper
1/8 tsp oregano seasoning
Directions:
Heat the air fryer to the temperature of 380°F.
Cut the ends off the sweet potato and discard. Divide into 4 even pieces lengthwise.
Whisk the avocado oil and all of the seasonings until combined thoroughly.
Brush the spices on top of the slices of sweet potato.
Transfer the slices to the air fryer basket and fry for 15 minutes.
Turn the sweet potato pieces over and steam once again for 15 more minutes.
Remove to a serving plate and enhance with your preferred toppings.
Nutrition:
Calories: 56
Carbs: 13g
Fat: 0g
Protein: 1g

30. Tomato Mushroom Frittata

Preparation time: 15 minutes
Cooking time: 15 minutes
Servings: 4
Ingredients:
2 tbsp skim milk
1/8 tsp pepper
2 tbsp chives, chopped
1/4 cup tomato, sliced
8 oz egg whites
1/4 cup mushrooms, sliced
Directions:
Adjust the air fryer to 320°F.
Using a glass dish, blend the tomato, egg whites, mushrooms, and milk until combined.
Incorporate the seasonings of chives and pepper into the mixture.
Empty into the skillet and warm for about 15 minutes.
Serve immediately and enjoy while hot.
Nutrition:
Calories: 303
Carbs: 4g
Fat: 19g
Protein: 26g

31. Ham, Spinach, and Egg in a Cup

Preparation time: 15 minutes
Cooking time: 8 minutes
Servings: 4
Ingredients:
4 eggs
4 thick slices of deli ham
4 tablespoons of spinach, chopped
Black pepper, to taste
4 tablespoons of cheddar cheese, shredded
Directions:
Grease 4 muffin tins and put the ham slices in it.
Press the muffin tins into cups gently.
Stir in the spinach and cheddar cheese. Top with the eggs and keep aside.

Set on an Air fryer to 375 degrees F for 8 minutes.
Serve.
Nutrition:
Calories: 228
Protein: 17.2g
Carbs: 6.6g
Fat: 15.6g

32. Yummy Breakfast Frittata

Preparation time: 15 minutes
Cooking time: 14 minutes
Servings: 2
Ingredients:
6 fresh mushrooms, sliced
6 cherry tomatoes, halved
½ cup of Parmesan cheese, grated and divided
1 bacon slice, chopped
3 eggs
1 tablespoon of olive oil
Salt and black pepper, to taste
Directions:
Combine mushrooms with tomatoes, bacon, salt, and black pepper in a bowl. Place the mushroom mixture on the cooking tray.
Set the air fryer oven to 390 degrees F for 6 minutes. Now, whisk eggs with Parmesan cheese and pour over the mushroom mixture. Cook again in the air fryer oven for about 8 minutes and dish out to serve.
Nutrition:
Calories: 397
Protein: 27.3g
Carbs: 17.8g
Fat: 26.2g

33. Sausage Bacon Beans Cancan

Preparation time: 15 minutes
Cooking time: 20 minutes
Servings: 6
Ingredients:
6 medium sausages
6 bacon slices
4 eggs
6 bread slices, toasted
1 can of baked beans
Salt and pepper, to taste
Directions:
Place the bacon and sausages in the cooking tray. Set the air fryer oven to 350 degrees F for 10 minutes.
Beat the eggs with salt and black pepper and pour in a ramekin.
Put the baked beans in another ramekin. Transfer both the ramekins in the air fryer oven and cook for about 10 minutes.
Divide the sausage mixture, bread slices, eggs, and beans in serving plates to serve.
Nutrition:
Calories: 518
Protein: 29.9g
Carbs: 20g
Fat: 34.9g

34. Bacon and Eggs in a Cup

Preparation time: 15 minutes
Cooking time: 16 minutes
Servings: 2
Ingredients:
2 bread slices, toasted and buttered
½ teaspoon of red pepper
1 teaspoon of marinara sauce
1 bacon slice
2 eggs
2 tablespoons of milk
1 tablespoon of Parmesan cheese, grated
Freshly ground black pepper, to taste
Directions:
Place the bacon in the cooking tray, set in the Air fryer to 355 degrees F for 8 minutes.
Chop the bacon into tiny pieces and divide it into 2 ramekins. Crack 1 egg in each ramekin over bacon and drizzle evenly with milk.
Top with marinara sauce and Parmesan cheese. Season with black pepper and place the ramekins in the air fryer. Cook for about 8 minutes and dish out to serve.
Nutrition:
Calories: 186
Protein: 13.2g
Carbs: 6.8g
Fat: 11.7g

35. Crispy Bread Rolls

Preparation time: 15 minutes
Cooking time: 18 minutes
Servings: 4
Ingredients:
8 bread slices, trimmed
5 large potatoes, boiled and mashed
2 small onions, chopped finely
2 green chilies, seeded and chopped finely
2 tablespoons of fresh cilantro, chopped finely
½ teaspoon of ground turmeric
½ teaspoon of mustard seeds
1 teaspoon of curry powder
Salt, to taste
2 tablespoons of olive oil, divided
Directions:
Put 1 tablespoon of olive oil along with mustard seeds in a large skillet on medium heat, sauté for about 30 seconds
Add onions, curry leaves, turmeric, sauté for about 5 minutes and stir in the mashed potatoes. Season with salt and mix thoroughly.
Dish out in a bowl and fold in the chilies and cilantro. Make 8 equal-sized patties out of this mixture.
Moisten the bread slices and then gently squeeze with your palms.
Place each patty in the center of each moistened bread slice and fold the bread entirely around the patty. Arrange the rolls in the cooking tray and drizzle with the remaining olive oil.
Arrange Air fryer to 390 degrees F for 13 minutes.
Serve warm with tea.
Nutrition:
Calories: 445
Protein: 9.7g
Carbs: 85.5g
Fat: 8.1g

36. Colorful Hash Brown

Preparation time: 15 minutes
Cooking time: 25 minutes
Servings: 2
Ingredients:
½ green bell pepper, seeded and chopped
½ tablespoon of extra-virgin olive oil
¼ tablespoon of dried oregano, crushed
¼ tablespoon of garlic powder
¼ tablespoon of red chili powder
½ red bell pepper, seeded and chopped
¼ tablespoon of ground cumin
½ onion, chopped
½ jalapeño, chopped
Salt and black pepper, to taste
5 russet potatoes, peeled, cubed, and soaked in water for 30 minutes
Directions:
Combine potatoes with olive oil in a bowl and place it in the cooking tray.
Set air fryer to 390 degrees F for 5 minutes. Mash the potatoes along with the rest of the ingredients and place them in the cooking tray.
Insert in the air fryer oven and cook again for about 20 minutes. Dish out in a plate and serve warm.
Nutrition:
Calories: 220
Protein: 5.2g
Carbs: 46g
Fat: 2.3g

37. Delish Mushroom Frittata

Preparation time: 15 minutes
Cooking time: 17 minutes
Servings: 2
Ingredients:
Cooking spray, as required
3 tablespoons of feta cheese, crumbled
1 tablespoon of olive oil
3 eggs
Salt, to taste
½ red onion, sliced thinly
2 cups of button mushrooms, sliced thinly
Directions:
Put olive oil, onion, and mushrooms in a skillet on medium heat. Sauté for about 5 minutes and dish out the mixture in a bowl.
Whisk the eggs with salt in a bowl and pour it into the ramekin. Top with the mushroom mixture and feta cheese.
Arrange the ramekins in the cooking tray, set in the Air fryer to 360 degrees F for 12 minutes. Serve with bread slices.
Nutrition:
Calories: 220
Protein: 12.8g
Carbs: 6g
Fat: 17.1g

38. Supreme Breakfast Burrito

Preparation time: 15 minutes
Cooking time: 8 minutes
Servings: 2
Ingredients:
2 eggs
2 tablespoons of salsa
2 whole-wheat tortillas
4-ounces of chicken breast slices, cooked
¼ of avocado, peeled, pitted, and sliced
2 tablespoons of mozzarella cheese, grated
Salt and black pepper, to taste
Directions:
Beat the eggs with salt plus black pepper in a bowl.
Transfer the whisked eggs into a nonstick pan and place it in the cooking tray.
Set "Air fryer" to 390 degrees F for 5 minutes.
Arrange the tortillas on a plate and divide the eggs, chicken slice, and avocado among the tortillas.
Top with salsa and mozzarella cheese and tightly roll each tortilla. Set "Air fryer" again to 355 degrees F for 3 minutes. Serve.
Nutrition:
Calories: 281
Protein: 26.2g
Carbs: 15.4g
Fat: 13g

39. Fluffy Cheesy Omelet

Preparation time: 15 minutes
Cooking time: 5 minutes
Servings: 2
Ingredients:
1 large onion, sliced
4 eggs
1/8 cup of cheddar cheese, grated
Cooking spray
1/8 cup of mozzarella cheese, grated
ground black pepper, to taste
¼ teaspoon of soy sauce
Directions:
Whisk eggs, black pepper, and soy sauce in a bowl.
Arrange the onions in the cooking tray and top with the egg mixture and cheese.
Set Air fryer to 360 degrees F for 5 minutes. Serve warm.
Nutrition:
Calories: 216
Protein: 15.5g
Carbs: 7.9g
Fat: 13.8g

40. Protein-Rich Breakfast

Preparation time: 15 minutes
Cooking time: 23 minutes
Servings: 4
Ingredients:
7-ounces of ham, sliced
4 teaspoons of milk
1 tablespoon of olive oil
1 tablespoon of unsalted butter, melted
1 pound of fresh baby spinach
4 eggs
Salt and black pepper, to taste
Directions:
Put olive oil and spinach in a skillet on medium heat. Sauté for about 3 minutes and drain the spinach

thoroughly. Transfer this spinach into the ramekins and layer with ham slices.
Crack 1 egg into each ramekin over ham slices and pour in the milk. Sprinkle with salt and black pepper and place in the cooking tray.
Set Air fryer to 355 degrees F for 20 minutes. Serve hot.

Nutrition:
Calories: 228
Protein: 17.2g
Carbs: 6.6g
Fat: 15.8g

41. Egg in a Bread Basket

Preparation time: 15 minutes
Cooking time: 10 minutes
Servings: 2

Ingredients:
2 bread slices
2 eggs
½ tablespoon of olive oil
1/8 teaspoon of maple syrup
1/8 teaspoon of balsamic vinegar
¼ teaspoon of fresh parsley, chopped
Salt and black pepper, to taste
2 tablespoons of mayonnaise
1 bacon slice, chopped
4 tomato slices
1 tablespoon of Mozzarella cheese, shredded

Directions:
Grease 2 ramekins and arrange 1 bread slice in each ramekin. Add tomato and bacon slices and sprinkle with the Mozzarella cheese.
Put 1 egg into each ramekin and pour in the balsamic vinegar and maple syrup. Sprinkle with parsley, salt, and black pepper and place in the cooking tray.
Set Air fryer to 325 degrees F for 10 minutes. Top with mayonnaise and serve hot.

Nutrition:
Calories: 245
Protein: 12.8 g
Carbs: 10.2g
Fat: 17.1g

42. Tasty Egg Yolks with Squid

Preparation time: 15 minutes
Cooking time: 16 minutes
Servings: 4

Ingredients:
4 raw salted egg yolks
2 tablespoons of evaporated milk
½ cup of chicken broth
½ cup of self-rising flour
14-ounces of flower squid, cleaned and dried

1 tablespoon of sugar
2 green chilies, seeded and chopped
3 tablespoons of olive oil
1 tablespoon of curry powder
Salt and black pepper, to taste

Directions:
Coat the flower squid with flour and season with salt and black pepper. Place the flower squid in the cooking tray. Set Air fryer to 375 degrees F for 8 minutes.
Remove and then put olive oil, chilies, and curry leaves in a skillet on medium heat. Sauté for about 3 minutes and whisk in the egg yolks and chicken broth.
Cook for about 5 minutes, continuously stirring, and fold in the evaporated milk and sugar. Combine well and add the fried flower squid. Toss until coated evenly and serve hot.

Nutrition:
Calories: 311
Protein: 21g
Carbs: 19.8g
Fat: 16.1g

43. Sweet Mustard Balls

Preparation time: 15 minutes
Cooking time: 15 minutes
Servings: 4

Ingredients:
1 teaspoon of mustard
1 teaspoon of honey
½ pound of ground pork
1 onion, chopped
2 tablespoons of fresh basil, chopped
½ tablespoon of Parmesan cheese, grated
1 teaspoon of garlic paste
Salt and black pepper, to taste
½ tablespoon of cheddar cheese, grated

Directions:
Mingle all the ingredients in a bowl and make equal-sized balls from the mixture. Place the balls on the cooking tray.
Set Air fryer to 395 degrees F for 15 minutes. Serve hot.

Nutrition:
Calories: 110
Protein: 15.9g
Carbs: 4.6g
Fat: 2.9g

44. Cherry Tomato Frittata

Preparation time: 15 minutes
Cooking time: 10 minutes
Servings: 2

Ingredients:
3 eggs
1 tablespoon of Parmesan cheese, shredded
1 teaspoon of fresh parsley, chopped
1 tablespoon of olive oil
½ of Italian sausage
4 cherry tomatoes, halved
Salt and black pepper, to taste

Directions:
Arrange the sausage and tomatoes in the cooking tray.
Set Air fryer to 360 degrees F for 5 minutes, then remove. Whisk eggs with Parmesan cheese, parsley, oil, salt, and black pepper in a bowl.
Pour the egg mixture over the sausage mixture and place it in the cooking tray. Set Air fryer again to 360 degrees F for 5 minutes. Serve warm.

Nutrition:

Calories: 293
Protein: 16.8g
Carbs: 10.4g
Fat: 21.5g

45. Spanish Style Frittata

Preparation time: 15 minutes
Cooking time: 11 minutes
Servings: 2

Ingredients:

3 jumbo eggs
1 tablespoon of olive oil
½ cup of frozen corn
½ of chorizo sausage, sliced
1 potato, boiled, peeled, and cubed
2 tablespoons of feta cheese, crumbled
Salt and black pepper, to taste

Directions:

Put the chorizo sausage, corn, and potato in a cooking tray greased with olive oil.
Set Air fryer to 355 degrees F for 6 minutes, and remove. Whisk the eggs with salt and black pepper in a bowl.
Drizzle this mixture over the sausage mixture and sprinkle with feta cheese. Place in the air fryer oven and cook for about 5 minutes. Dish out on a plate and serve with toast.

Nutrition:

Calories: 327
Protein: 15.3g
Carbs: 23.3g
Fat: 20.2g

46. Cheesy Garlic Sweet Potatoes

Preparation time: 15 minutes
Cooking time: 40 minutes
Servings: 8

Ingredients:

¼ cup garlic butter, melted
4 sweet potatoes, halved lengthwise
¾ cup Mozzarella cheese, shredded
½ cup Parmesan cheese, grated
2 tablespoons parsley, chopped
Sea salt and black pepper, to taste

Directions:

Brush potatoes with garlic butter and season well with salt and pepper. Place cut side down on a greased baking pan.
Set the temperature to 425 F and the time to 30 minutes on the air fryer oven.
Remove, flip and top with parsley, mozzarella and parmesan.
Set the temperature to Broil and the time to 2 minutes. Season well and serve.

Nutrition:

Calories 162
Fat 9 g
Carbs 5 g
Protein 5 g

47. Blueberry Muffins

Preparation time: 15 minutes
Cooking time: 20 minutes
Servings: 12

Ingredients:

1 egg
1 cup + 1 tablespoon all-purpose flour, unbleached
1 ½ teaspoons baking powder
4 tablespoons unsalted butter
¾ cup granulated sugar
¼ cup whole milk
½ teaspoon pure vanilla extract
1 cup blueberries, fresh
¼ teaspoon kosher salt
Pinch ground cinnamon
Cooking spray

Directions:

Add baking powder, 1 cup flour, salt, and cinnamon into a bowl. Whisk to combine well.
Add sugar and butter into a bowl. Mix until creamy, then add vanilla extract and egg and mix to combine well. Add milk and stir well.
Mix dry fixing with wet fixing. Stir well to combine.
Mix blueberries with 1 tablespoon flour and add to the batter. Combine.
Grease a 6 cups muffin tray with cooking spray. Add the mixture to the tin.
Bake in the air fryer oven, set the temperature to 325 F, and 20 minutes. Serve.

Nutrition:

Calories 269
Fat 10 g
Carbs 17 g
Protein 15 g

48. Eggs, Bacon, Tomato and Cheese Bake

Preparation time: 15 minutes
Cooking time: 1 hour & 40 minutes
Servings: 8

Ingredients:

¼ cup extra-virgin olive oil
1 lb. bakery white bread, cut into 1" cubes
1 onion, halved and sliced
1 lb. sliced applewood-smoked bacon, cut into ½" pieces
28 oz. can whole Italian tomatoes, chopped
½ lb. extra-sharp cheddar, shredded
½ teaspoon red pepper, crushed
½ lb. Monterey Jack cheese, shredded
2 tablespoons snipped chives
1 ¾ cups chicken broth
8 eggs
Salt, to taste

Directions:

Grease a baking dish with cooking spray. Toss bread with olive oil in a bowl and arrange on a baking pan.
Set the air fryer oven temperature to 350 F and the time to 20 minutes, tossing twice.
Cook bacon in a skillet for 8 minutes over high heat. Drain the bacon and reserve 2 tablespoons fat in the skillet.
Put the onions to the skillet and cook for 5 minutes over medium heat. Add crushed red pepper and tomatoes and cook for 3 minutes.
Add the toasted bread cubes back to the bowl, then the skillet contents along with shredded cheeses, bacon, broth, and chives. Stir well—season with salt.

Put, and spread the batter in the baking dish, bake in the air fryer oven.
Set to 350 F and the time to 45 minutes.
Remove and make 8 wells in the bread mixture.
Crack an egg into each well and return the dish to the air fryer oven—Bake for 15 minutes. Serve.
Nutrition:
Calories 953
Fat 57.9 g
Carbs 61 g
Protein 47 g

49. Strawberry-Almond Scones

Preparation time: 15 minutes
Cooking time: 1 hour & 45 minutes
Servings: 16
Ingredients:
1 ½ cups whole wheat pastry flour
1 ½ cups all-purpose flour
1 tablespoon baking powder
¼ cup + 2 tablespoons granulated sugar
½ teaspoon baking soda
1 stick unsalted butter, cold, cubed
1 ¼ cups buttermilk
1 ½ cups strawberries, sliced
2 tablespoons turbinado sugar
½ teaspoon salt
2 cups confectioners' sugar
½ cup almonds, sliced, toasted
3 tablespoons buttermilk
½ teaspoon almond extract
Pinch of salt
Directions:
Mix all-purpose flour and whole wheat pastry flour in a bowl with baking powder, granulated sugar, baking soda, and ½ teaspoon salt.
Add the butter and stir until the mixture resembles a coarse meal. Add 1 ¼ cups buttermilk and add sliced strawberries.
Shape the dough into the scones and place them on the baking pan. Brush cones with buttermilk and add turbinado sugar on top.
Set re to 400 F and the time to 35 minutes. Let cool on the rack for 30 minutes.
Adjust the oven temperature to 350 F.
Whisk confectioners' sugar, almond extract, buttermilk, and salt in a bowl. Cover and let rest.
Add glaze on top of the scones then top with almonds. Let dry for 10 minutes. Serve.
Nutrition:
Calories 153
Fat 0.7 g
Carbs 34 g
Protein 4 g

50. Spinach-Egg Breakfast Pizzas

Preparation time: 15 minutes
Cooking time: 17 minutes
Servings: 4
Ingredients:
1 tablespoon olive oil
1 lb. frozen pizza dough, thawed
6 oz. baby spinach
3 tablespoons sour cream
1/3 cup Parmesan cheese
1 garlic clove, minced
4 large eggs
¼ teaspoon of sea salt
1/8 teaspoon black pepper
Cornmeal
Directions:
Sprinkle a baking pan with cornmeal. Slice dough into 4 pieces, then shapes into 7" circles and place on a pan.
Heat 1 tablespoon oil in a skillet over medium heat. Add spinach and cook for 2 minutes.
Mix spinach with cheese, sour cream, garlic clove, salt, and pepper. Add spinach mixture over each pizza.
Set the temperature to 450 F and the time to 5 minutes.
Remove and add an egg to the center of each pizza. Bake again within 10 minutes. Season with pepper. Serve.
Nutrition:
Calories 433
Fat 14 g
Carbs 55 g
Protein 16 g

51. Amish Baked Oatmeal

Preparation time: 15 minutes
Cooking time: 30 minutes
Servings: 6
Ingredients:
½ cup milk
½ cup of sugar
1 ½ cups quick-cooking oats
1 teaspoon baking soda
¼ cup butter, melted
1 egg
1 teaspoon vanilla extract
¾ teaspoon salt
Warm milk
Directions:
Put all the fixing in a bowl except milk and mix well.
Add to a greased baking pan.
Set the temperature of the air fryer oven to 350 F and the time to 30 minutes. Serve.
Nutrition:
Calories 235
Fat 10 g
Carbs 31 g
Protein 5 g

52. Mixed Berry Toast Bake

Preparation time: 15 minutes
Cooking time: 50 minutes
Servings: 8
Ingredients:
1 ¾ cups of fat-free milk
6 eggs
1 teaspoon ground cinnamon
1 teaspoon sugar
1 teaspoon vanilla extract
1 French loaf bread, cubed
2 tablespoons cold butter
12 oz. frozen unsweetened mixed berries

1/3 cup packed brown sugar
¼ teaspoon salt

Directions:

Whisk milk, eggs, cinnamon, sugar, vanilla extract, and salt in a bowl. Grease a baking pan using a cooking spray and add bread cubes on it. Refrigerate overnight.

Remove berries and French toast from the fridge and let rest for 10 minutes.

Set to 350 F and the time to 30 minutes.

Cut butter and add to brown sugar to a bowl. Add berries to French toast and sprinkle with brown sugar mixture. Bake again for 20 minutes. Serve.

Nutrition:

Calories 310
Fat 8 g
Carbs 46 g
Protein 13 g

53. Bananas Foster French Toast

Preparation time: 15 minutes
Cooking time: 40 minutes
Servings: 6

Ingredients:

3 bananas, sliced
½ cup butter, cubed
2/3 cup packed brown sugar
½ teaspoon ground cinnamon
½ cup heavy whipping cream
½ teaspoon ground allspice
12 slices egg bread
3 eggs
1 ½ cups 2% milk
1 tablespoon sugar
1 teaspoon vanilla extract

Directions:

Add butter to a heat-proof bowl, cover, and microwave for 45 seconds. Add cream, sugar, cinnamon, and allspice. Add bananas and toss gently. Transfer to a greased baking pan. Add bread on top. Add the rest of the ingredients to a blender. Process until well combined and add over the bread. Refrigerate overnight.

Set the temperature to 375 F and the time to 40 minutes. Let rest for 10 minutes. Serve.

Nutrition:

Calories 658
Fat 31 g
Carbs 84 g
Protein 14 g

54. Fruity Baked Oatmeal

Preparation time: 15 minutes
Cooking time: 40 minutes
Servings: 9

Ingredients:

2 eggs, lightly beaten
3 cups quick-coating oats
1 cup packed brown sugar
2 teaspoons baking powder
½ teaspoon ground cinnamon
1 cup fat-free milk
¾ cup tart apple, peeled and chopped
½ cup butter, melted
1/3 cup peaches, chopped
1/3 cup blueberries
1 teaspoon salt

Directions:

Mix brown sugar, oats, baking powder, cinnamon, and salt in a bowl. Mix milk, eggs, plus butter in a separate bowl and add to the dry ingredients. Add peaches, apple, and blueberries.

Add the mixture to a baking dish coated with cooking spray.

Bake in the air fryer oven with a temperature of 350 F and the time to 40 minutes.

Cut into squares. Serve.

Nutrition:

Calories 322
Fat 13 g
Carbs 46 g
Protein 7 g

55. Pumpkin French Toast Casserole

Preparation time: 15 minutes
Cooking time: 70 minutes
Servings: 12

Ingredients:

8 eggs
1 loaf cinnamon-raisin bread
8 oz. reduced-fat cream cheese, cut into ¾" cubes
1 cup canned pumpkin
12 oz. evaporated milk
½ cup fat-free milk
2/3 cup packed brown sugar
¼ teaspoon ground nutmeg
2 teaspoons ground cinnamon
¼ teaspoon ground ginger
1/8 teaspoon ground cloves
½ cup pecans, chopped
½ teaspoon salt

Directions:

Cut each bread slice into quarters. Put half of the bread into a greased baking dish. Top with cubed cream cheese and remaining bread.

Whisk evaporated milk, eggs, pumpkin, brown sugar, fat-free milk, spices, and salt in a bowl. Pour over the dish. Refrigerate overnight, covered.

Select the Bake setting. Set to 350 F and the time to 40 minutes.

Add pecans—Bake for 30 minutes. Let rest for 10 minutes. Serve.

Nutrition:

Calories 302
Fat 13 g
Carbs 36 g
Protein 13 g

56. Chorizo Egg Casserole

Preparation time: 15 minutes
Cooking time: 70 minutes
Servings: 8

Ingredients:

3 cups hash brown potatoes, frozen and cubed
1 lb. fresh chorizo
1 medium onion, diced
2 garlic cloves, minced
¾ cup sweet red pepper, chopped

[illegible] eggs
4 oz. can chop green chilies
1 ½ cups half-and-half cream
2 teaspoons chili powder
1 cup cheddar cheese, shredded
1 cup Monterey Jack cheese, shredded
3 tablespoons cilantro, minced

Directions:

Crumble and cook chorizo in a skillet over medium-high heat for 7 minutes. Drain well.

Cook onion, potatoes, and pepper in the skillet for 7 minutes, then add garlic and cook for 1 minute. Remove from heat and add chorizo—Cook for 15 minutes.

Whisk green chilies, eggs, cream, and chili powder in a bowl. Add half of the chorizo mixture, cheeses, and egg mixture to a greased baking dish and spread well. Add 1 tablespoon cilantro on top. Top with remaining eggs and chorizo. Add remaining cheese and 1 tablespoon cilantro. Refrigerate overnight.

Set the air fryer oven to 350 F and the time to 40 minutes.

Let rest for 10 minutes. Add remaining cilantro on top. Serve.

Nutrition:

Calories 461
Fat 34 g
Carbs 10 g
Protein 25 g

57. Hacienda Hash Browns

Preparation time: 15 minutes
Cooking time: 60 minutes
Servings: 8

Ingredients:

1 onion, chopped
2 tablespoons butter
1 red pepper, chopped
1 garlic clove, minced
6 eggs
1 ¼ cups tortilla chips, crushed
3 tablespoons cilantro, minced
½ teaspoon ground cumin
1 2/3 cups cheddar cheese, shredded
6 cups hash brown potatoes, thawed and shredded
1 cup 4% cottage cheese
2/3 cup canned black beans, rinsed and drained
½ cup pepper jack cheese, shredded
½ teaspoon salt
¼ teaspoon pepper

Directions:

Heat butter in a skillet over medium heat. Add red pepper and onion and cook for 4 minutes. Add garlic and cook for 1 minute. Remove from heat and let it cool.

Add ¾ cup crushed tortilla chips to a greased baking dish. Whisk eggs, cumin, cilantro, salt, and pepper in a bowl.

Add hash browns, cottage cheese, 1 cup cheddar cheese, black beans, onion mixture, and pepper jack cheese. Add over the chips.

Set to 350 F and the time to 45 minutes.

Add remaining tortilla chips and cheddar cheese on top—Bake for 10 minutes. Serve.

Nutrition:

Calories 341
Fat 20 g
Carbs 24 g
Protein 18 g

58. Peach French Toast

Preparation time: 15 minutes
Cooking time: 60 minutes
Servings: 6

Ingredients:

5 eggs
1 ½ cups whole milk
1 cup packed brown sugar
½ cup butter, cubed
2 tablespoons water
1 tablespoon vanilla extract
12 slices day-old French bread
29 oz. can slice peaches, drained
Ground cinnamon

Directions:

Add butter, water, and brown sugar to a pan and bring to boil. Reduce the heat and simmer for 10 minutes, stirring often. Add to a greased baking dish and add peaches on top. Add bread over the peaches.

Whisk milk, eggs, and vanilla in a bowl and pour over the bread. Cover and refrigerate overnight.

Remove the dish 30 minutes before baking. Add cinnamon on top.

Set the air fryer oven to 350 F and the time to 50 minutes. Serve.

Nutrition:

Calories 607
Fat 26.8 g
Carbs 79 g
Protein 14 g

59. Ham Strata

Preparation time: 15 minutes
Cooking time: 35 minutes
Servings: 8

Ingredients:

2 onions, quartered and sliced
1 teaspoon olive oil
¾ cup green pepper, julienned
¾ cup sweet red pepper, julienned
1 loaf French bread, cut into ½" cubes
1 cup Monterey Jack cheese, shredded
1 ½ cups fully cooked ham, cubed
6 eggs
2 cups 2% milk
¼ teaspoon salt
½ teaspoon pepper

Directions:

Heat-up oil in a skillet over medium-high heat. Cook peppers and onion until tender. Grease a baking pan with cooking spray.

Layer half of onion mixture, bread cubes, ham, and cheese on it. Repeat layers.

Whisk milk, eggs, pepper, and salt and add over the layers. Refrigerate overnight.

Set the air fryer oven temperature to 350 F and the time to 35 minutes. Serve.

Nutrition:

Calories 393
Fat 16 g
Carbs 38 g
Protein 23 g

60. Hash Brown Maple Sausage Casserole

Preparation time: 15 minutes
Cooking time: 60 minutes
Servings: 8

Ingredients:

2 tablespoons olive oil
1 lb. maple pork sausage
½ cup sweet potato, peeled and cubed
30 oz. pack frozen shredded hash brown potatoes, thawed
1 ½ cups Gruyere cheese, shredded
2 cups kale, chopped
5 large eggs, lightly beaten
¾ cup fresh corn
2 cups half-and-half cream
1 teaspoon salt
½ teaspoon pepper

Directions:

Cook sweet potato and sausage in a skillet over medium-high heat for 7 minutes and crumble well. Remove with a wooden spoon and drain.
Coat a skillet with oil—Reserve ½ cup hash browns for topping. Add the rest of the potatoes to the skillet. Press firmly to form an even layer.
Add layers of kale, cheese, and corn. Add hash browns and sausage mixture on top. Whisk cream, eggs, salt, and pepper in a bowl and add on top.
Bake in the air fryer oven to 375 F and the time to 55 minutes.
Let rest for 20 minutes. Serve.

Nutrition:

Calories 486
Fat 32 g
Carbs 27 g
Protein 22 g

Chapter 4. Poultry Recipes

61. Chicken Stir-Fry

Preparation Time: 10 minutes
Cooking Time: 20 minutes
Servings: 2

Ingredients:

1 (6-oz. chicken breast; cut into 1-inch cubes
½ medium red bell pepper; seeded and chopped
½ medium zucchini; chopped
¼ medium red onion; peeled and sliced
1 tbsp coconut oil
½ tsp garlic powder
1 tsp dried oregano
¼ tsp dried thyme

Directions:

Place all fixing into a large mixing bowl and toss until the coconut oil coats the meat and vegetables. Pour the contents of the bowl into the air fryer basket
Adjust the temperature to 375°F and set the timer for 15 minutes. Shake the fryer basket halfway through the cooking time to redistribute the food. Serve readily.

Nutrition:

Calories: 186
Protein: 20.4 g
Fiber: 1.7 g
Fat: 8.0 g
Carbohydrates: 5.6 g

62. Spiced Chicken Breasts

Preparation Time: 15 minutes
Cooking Time: 10 minutes
Servings: 4

Ingredients:

4 chicken breasts, skinless and boneless
1 tbsp. parsley; chopped
1 tsp. smoked paprika
1 tsp. garlic powder
1 tsp. chili powder
A drizzle of olive oil
A pinch of salt and black pepper

Directions:

Rub the chicken with salt plus pepper and rub it with the oil and all the other ingredients except the parsley
Put the chicken breasts in your air fryer's basket and cook at 350°F for 10 minutes on each side
Divide between plates, sprinkle the parsley on top and serve

Nutrition:

Calories: 222
Fat: 11 g
Fiber: 4 g
Carbohydrates: 6 g
Protein: 12 g

63. Nutmeg Chicken Thighs

Preparation Time: 15 minutes
Cooking Time: 20 minutes
Servings: 4

Ingredients:

2 lb. chicken thighs
2 tbsp. olive oil
½ tsp. nutmeg, ground
A pinch of salt and black pepper

Directions:

Massage the chicken thighs with salt and pepper and rub with the rest of the ingredients
Put the chicken thighs in the air fryer's basket, cook at 360°F for 15 minutes on each side, divide between plates and serve.

Nutrition:

Calories: 271
Fat: 12 g
Fiber: 4 g
Carbohydrates: 6 g
Protein: 13 g

64. Creamy Chicken Wings

Preparation Time: 5 minutes
Cooking Time: 30 minutes
Servings:

Ingredients:

2 lb. chicken wings
¼ cup parmesan, grated
½ cup heavy cream
3 garlic cloves; minced
3 tbsp butter; melted
½ tsp oregano; dried
½ tsp basil; dried
Salt and black pepper to taste.

Directions:

Mix the chicken wings with all the ingredients except the parmesan in a baking dish that fits your air fryer. Put the dish to your air fryer and cook at 380°F for 30 minutes. Sprinkle the cheese on top, leave the mix aside for 10 minutes, divide between plates and serve

Nutrition:

Calories: 270
Fat: 12 g
Fiber: 3 g
Carbohydrates: 6 g
Protein: 17 g

65. Turkey Turnovers

Preparation Time: 10 minutes
Cooking time: 10 minutes
Servings: 8

Ingredients:

2 cups turkey, cooked & chopped
1 cup cheddar cheese, grated
1 cup broccoli, cooked & chopped
½ cup mayonnaise
½ tsp. salt
¼ tsp. pepper
2 cans refrigerated crescent rolls

Directions:

Place the baking pan in position 1 of the oven.
In a large bowl, combine all ingredients, except rolls, mix well.
Separate each can of rolls into 4 squares, press perforations to seal.
Spoon turkey mixture in center of each square. Fold over diagonally and seal the edges.

Set the air fryer oven to "bake" at 375°F for 15 minutes.
Brush tops of turnovers lightly with additional mayonnaise. After the oven has preheated 5 minutes, place turnovers on baking pan and cook 10-12 minutes or until golden brown serve warm.

Nutrition:

Calories: 309
Fat: 21 g
Carbs: 15 g
Fiber: 2 g
Sugar: 1 g
Protein: 15 g

66. Chicken Parm

Preparation Time: 10 minutes
Cooking time: 35 minutes
Servings: 4

Ingredients:

Nonstick cooking spray
½ cup flour
2 eggs
2/3 cup panko breadcrumbs
2/3 cup Italian seasoned breadcrumbs
1/3 + ¼ cup parmesan cheese, divided
2 tbsp. fresh parsley, chopped
½ tsp. salt
¼ tsp. pepper
4 chicken breast halves, skinless & boneless
24 oz. marinara sauce
1 cup mozzarella cheese, grated

Directions:

Lightly spray your fryer basket with cooking spray. Place flour in a shallow dish.
In a separate shallow dish, beat the eggs.
In a third shallow dish, combine both breadcrumbs, 1/3 cup parmesan cheese, 2 tablespoons parsley, salt, and pepper.
Place chicken between two sheets of plastic wrap and pound to ½-inch thick.
Dip chicken first in flour, then eggs, and breadcrumb mixture to coat. Place in the basket and then put the basket on the baking pan.
Set oven to air fry at 375°F for 10 minutes. Flip the chicken over halfway through cooking time.
Remove chicken and baking pan from the oven. Place the rack in position 1. Set oven to bake at 425°F for 30 minutes.
Pour 1 ½ cups marinara in the bottom of an 8x11-inch baking dish. Place chicken over the sauce and add another 2 tablespoons marinara to tops of chicken. Top the chicken with mozzarella and parmesan cheese once oven preheats for 5 minutes, place the dish in the oven and bake 20-25 minutes until bubbly and cheese is golden brown. Serve.

Nutrition:

Calories: 529
Fat: 13 g
Sodium: 1437 mg
Carbs: 52 g
Fiber: 5 g
Sugar: 9 g
Protein: 51 g

67. Teriyaki Duck Legs

Preparation Time: 15 minutes
Cooking time: 2 hours
Servings: 6

Ingredients:

3 lbs. duck legs
½ cup teriyaki sauce
2 tbsp. soy sauce
2 tbsp. malt vinegar

Directions:

Place the rack in position 1 of the oven.
Place the duck legs, skin side up, in an 8x11-inch baking dish.
In a small bowl, whisk remaining fixing and pour around duck legs. The liquid needs to reach the skin level of duck, if not add water until it does.
Set the oven to convection bake at 300°F for 60 minutes. After 5 minutes, place the ducks in the oven and cook 90 minutes, or until tender.
Remove duck from the oven. Pour off cooking liquid into a small saucepan. Skim off fat and reserve. Bring sauce to a boil and cook until it reduces, about 10 minutes, stirring occasionally.
Place the duck legs in the fryer basket and brush with reserved fat and sauce. Place the basket in the oven and set to broil at 400°F for 10 minutes. Turn duck over halfway through and brush with fat and sauce again. Serve.

Nutrition:

Calories: 608
Fat: 20 g
Sodium: 1063 mg
Carbs: 6 g
Sugar: 5 g
Protein: 101 g

68. Turkey Burgers

Preparation Time: 10 minutes
Cooking time: 10 minutes
Servings: 4

Ingredients:

1 1/3 lb. ground turkey
½ cup gruyere cheese, grated
3 green onions, chopped fine
¼ cup breadcrumbs
¼ cup Dijon mustard
½ tsp. salt
½ tsp. pepper

Directions:

Mix all ingredients until a proper mixture is formed in a large bowl.
Form into 4 patties. Lightly spray tops with cooking spray and put them in the fryer basket, sprayed side down. Spray patties again.
Put the baking pan in position 2 of the air fryer oven and add the basket. Set oven to air fry at 400°F for 10 minutes. Turn burgers over halfway through cooking time. Serve.

Nutrition:

Calories: 321
Fat: 17 g
Sodium: 697 mg
Carbs: 7 g

Fiber: 1 g
Sugar: 1 g
Protein: 35 g

69. Korean Chicken Wings

Preparation Time: 5 minutes
Cooking time: 10 minutes
Servings: 8
Ingredients:
Wings:
1 tsp. pepper
1 tsp. salt
2 pounds of chicken wings
Sauce:
2 packets Splendid
1 tbsp minced garlic
1 tbsp minced ginger
1 tbsp sesame oil
1 tsp agave nectar
1 tbsp mayo
2 tbsp. gochujang
Finishing:
¼ cup green onions, chopped
2 tsp sesame seeds
Directions:
Make sure the air fryer oven is preheated to 400°. Place a rack onto the pan, line a small pan with foil, then place it into an air fryer oven.
Rub the wings with pepper plus salt and place onto the rack.
Set to 160°F and set time to 20 minutes and air fry 20 minutes, turning at 10 minutes.
As chicken air fries, mix all the sauce components.
Put half of the sauce mixture over wings, tossing well to coat.
Put coated wings back into the air fryer for 5 minutes or till they reach 165°.
Remove and sprinkle with green onions and sesame seeds. Dip into an extra sauce.
Nutrition:
Calories: 356
Fat: 26 g
Carbs: 0 g
Fiber: 0 g
Sugar: 2 g
Protein: 23 g

70. Almond Flour Coco-Milk Battered Chicken

Preparation Time: 5 minutes
Cooking time: 30 minutes
Servings: 35
Ingredients:
¼ cup of coconut milk
½ cup almond flour
1 ½ tablespoon old bay Cajun seasoning
1 egg, beaten
4 small chicken thighs
Salt and pepper to taste
Directions:
Preheat the air fryer oven for 5 minutes. Mix the egg and coconut milk in a bowl.
Soak the chicken thighs in the beaten egg mixture.
In a mixing bowl, combine the almond flour, Cajun seasoning, salt, and pepper.
Dredge the chicken thighs in the almond flour mixture.
Place in the air fryer basket. Cook for 30 minutes at 350°F.
Nutrition:
Calories: 590
Fat: 38 g
Carbs: 3.2 g
Fiber: 0 g
Sugar: 0 g
Protein: 32.5 g

71. Broccoli-Rice 'n Cheese Casserole

Preparation Time: 15 minutes
Cooking Time: 30 minutes
Servings: 4
Ingredients:
1 (10 ounces) can chunk chicken, drained
1 cup uncooked instant rice
1 cup of water
1/2 (10.75 ounces) can condense cream of chicken soup
1/2 (10.75 ounces) can condense cream of mushroom soup
1/2 cup milk
1/2 small white onion, chopped
1/2-pound processed cheese food
2 tablespoons butter
8-ounce frozen chopped broccoli
Directions:
Lightly grease baking pan of the air fryer with cooking spray. Put water and boil at 390°F. Mix in rice and cook for 3 minutes.
Stir in processed cheese, onion, broccoli, milk, butter, chicken soup, mushroom soup, and chicken. Mix well. Cook for 15 minutes at 390°F, fluff mixture, and continue cooking for another 10 minutes until tops are browned.
Serve and enjoy!
Nutrition:
Calories: 752
Carbs: 82.7 g
Protein: 36.0 g
Fat: 30.8 g

72. Buttered Spinach-Egg Omelet

Preparation Time: 15 minutes
Cooking Time: 15 minutes
Servings: 3
Ingredients:
¼ cup of coconut milk
1 tablespoon melted butter
1-pound baby spinach, chopped finely
3 tablespoons olive oil
4 eggs, beaten
Salt and pepper to taste
Directions:
Preheat the air fryer for 5 minutes.
In a mixing bowl, blend the eggs, coconut milk, olive oil, and butter until a fine mixture is formed.
Add the spinach and season with salt and pepper to taste.

Pour all ingredients in a baking dish that will fit in the air fryer.
Bake at 350°F for 15 minutes.

Nutrition:
Calories: 310
Carbohydrates: 3.6 g
Protein: 13.6 g
Fat: 26.8 g

73. Caesar Marinated Grilled Chicken

Preparation Time: 15 minutes
Cooking Time: 24 minutes
Servings: 3

Ingredients:
¼ cup crouton
1 teaspoon lemon zest. Form into ovals, skewer, and grill.
1/2 cup Parmesan
1/4 cup breadcrumbs
1-pound ground chicken
2 tablespoons Caesar dressing and more for drizzling
2-4 romaine leaves

Directions:
In a shallow dish, mix well chicken, 2 tablespoons Caesar dressing, parmesan, and breadcrumbs. Mix well with hands. Form into 1-inch oval patties.
Thread chicken pieces in skewers. Place on skewer rack in the air fryer.
For 12 minutes, cook at 360°F. Halfway through cooking time, turnover skewers. If needed, cook in batches.
Serve with croutons and extra dressing.

Nutrition:
Calories: 339
Carbs: 9.5 g
Protein: 32.6 g
Fat: 18.9 g

74. Cheese Stuffed Chicken

Preparation Time: 15 minutes
Cooking Time: 30 minutes
Servings: 10

Ingredients:
1 tablespoon creole seasoning
2 tablespoon olive oil
1/2teaspoon garlic powder
1/2 teaspoon onion powder
4 chicken breasts, butterflied and pounded
4 slices Colby cheese
4 slices pepper jack cheese

Directions:
Preheat the air fryer to 390°F.
Place the grill pan accessory in the air fryer.
Create the dry rub by mixing the creole seasoning, garlic powder, and onion powder in a bowl. Season with salt and pepper if desired.
Rub the seasoning on to the chicken.
Place the chicken on a working surface and slice each of the pepper jack and Colby cheese.
Fold the chicken and secure the edges with toothpicks.
Brush chicken with olive oil.
Grill for 30 minutes and make sure to flip the meat every 10 minutes.

Nutrition:
Calories: 727
Carbs: 5.4 g
Protein: 73.1 g
Fat: 45.9 g

75. Bacon-Wrapped Chicken Breasts

Preparation time: 15 minutes
Cooking time: 14 minutes
Servings: 2

Ingredients:
2 chicken breasts
8 oz onion and chive cream cheese
1 tbsp butter
6 turkey bacon
Salt to taste
1 tbsp fresh parsley, chopped
Juice from ½ lemon

Directions:
Preheat on Air Fry to 390 F. Stretch out the bacon slightly and lay them in 2 sets; 3 bacon strips on each side. Place the chicken breast on each bacon set and use a knife to smear cream cheese on both.
Share the butter on top and sprinkle with salt. Cover the bacon around the chicken and secure the ends into the wrap. Place the wrapped chicken in the basket and press Start.
Cook for 14 minutes. Remove the chicken onto a serving platter and top with parsley and lemon juice. Serve with steamed greens.

Nutrition:
Calories: 530
Carbs: 0g
Fat: 0g
Protein: 0g

76. Sweet Asian Chicken Wings

Preparation time: 15 minutes
Cooking time: 15 minutes
Servings: 6

Ingredients:
1 lb. chicken wings
1 cup flour
1 cup breadcrumbs
2 eggs, beaten
2 tbsp canola oil
Salt and black pepper to taste
2 tbsp sesame seeds
2 tbsp Korean red pepper paste
1 tbsp apple cider vinegar
2 tbsp honey
1 tbsp soy sauce

Directions:
Preheat air fryer oven to 390 F. Separates the chicken wings into winglets and drumettes. In a bowl, mix oil, salt, and pepper.
Coat chicken with flour, followed by eggs and breadcrumbs. Place it in the basket. Spray with a bit of oil and press Start—Cook for 15 minutes.
Mix red pepper paste, apple cider vinegar, soy sauce, honey, and ¼ cup water in a saucepan over medium heat and bring the mixture to a boil.
Add in the chicken and toss to coat. Garnish with sesame seeds and serve.

Nutrition:
Calories: 176
Carbs: 6g
Fat: 12g
Protein: 12g

77. Paprika Chicken Breasts with Ham & Cheese

Preparation time: 15 minutes
Cooking time: 21 minutes
Servings: 4
Ingredients:
4 chicken breasts
4 ham slices
4 Swiss cheese slices
3 tbsp all-purpose flour
4 tbsp butter
1 tbsp paprika
1 tbsp chicken bouillon granules
½ cup dry white wine
1 cup heavy whipping cream
1 tbsp cornstarch
Directions:
Preheat the air fryer oven to 380 F. Pound the chicken breasts and put a slice of ham on each of the chicken breasts. Fold the edges over the filling and close with toothpicks.
In a bowl, combine paprika and flour and coat in the chicken. Press Start and fry the chicken for 14-16 minutes.
Melt the butter in a skillet and add the bouillon and wine. Stir to combine and reduce the heat to low. Transfer the chicken from the oven and place it in the skillet. Let simmer for 5 minutes.
Nutrition:
Calories: 248
Carbs: 3g
Fat: 13g
Protein: 30g

78. Chili Chicken Strips with Aioli

Preparation time: 15 minutes
Cooking time: 14 minutes
Servings: 4
Ingredients:
1 lb. chicken breasts, cut into strips
2 tbsp olive oil
1 cup breadcrumbs
½ tbsp garlic powder
½ tbsp chili powder
½ cup mayonnaise
Directions
Preheat the air fryer oven to 350 F. Mix breadcrumbs, garlic powder, and chili on a plate. Coat the strips in the breadcrumb mixture. Drizzle with olive oil.
Arrange the chicken strips on the basket and press Start—Cook for 12-14 minutes.
To prepare the aioli: combine mayo with ground chili. Serve with the chicken strips.
Nutrition:
Calories: 281
Carbs: 24g
Fat: 7g
Protein: 39g

79. Cheesy Chicken with Tomato Sauce

Preparation time: 15 minutes
Cooking time: 10 minutes
Servings: 2
Ingredients:
2 chicken breasts, ½-inch thick
1 egg, beaten
½ cup breadcrumbs
Salt and black pepper to taste
2 tbsp tomato sauce
2 tbsp Grana Padano cheese, grated
¼ cup mozzarella cheese, shredded
Directions:
Preheat the air fryer oven to 350 F. Dip the breasts into the egg, then into the crumbs, and arrange on the greased basket.
Cook for 5 minutes. Turn, drizzle with tomato sauce, sprinkle with Grana Padano and mozzarella cheeses, and cook for 5 more minutes. Serve warm.
Nutrition:
Calories: 120
Carbs: 5g
Fat: 4g
Protein: 16g

80. Crunchy Chicken Tenderloins

Preparation time: 15 minutes
Cooking time: 14 minutes
Servings: 4
Ingredients:
8 chicken tenderloins
2 tbsp butter, melted
2 oz breadcrumbs
1 large egg, whisked
Directions
Preheat the air fryer oven to 380 F. Dip the chicken in the egg.
Then roll up them the crumbs. Drizzle with melted butter and arrange on the frying basket.
Press Start and cook for 12-14 minutes. Set to Broil function for crispier taste. Serve warm.
Nutrition:
Calories: 100
Carbs: 0g
Fat: 1g
Protein: 23g

81. Homemade Tarragon Chicken

Preparation time: 15 minutes
Cooking time: 15 minutes
Servings: 4
Ingredients:
1 lb. chicken breasts
½ tbsp butter, melted
Salt and black pepper to taste
¼ tsp dried tarragon
Directions
Preheat your air fryer oven on Bake function to 380 F. Place each chicken breast on a 12x12 inches foil. Drizzle with butter and sprinkle with tarragon, salt, and pepper.

Wrap the foil around the chicken loosely to create an airflow—Bake for 15 minutes. Carefully unwrap and serve.

Nutrition:
Calories: 275
Carbs: 6g
Fat: 11g
Protein: 31g

82. Sweet Sticky Chicken Wings

Preparation time: 15 minutes
Cooking time: 15 minutes
Servings: 4

Ingredients:
16 chicken wings
¼ cup butter
¼ cup honey
½ tbsp salt
4 garlic cloves, minced
¾ cup potato starch

Directions:
Preheat air fryer oven to 370 F. Coat the wings with potato starch and place them in a greased baking dish. Press Start and cook for 5 minutes.
Mix the rest of the fixing in a bowl. Pour the sauce over the wings and cook for another 10 minutes. Serve warm.

Nutrition:
Calories: 230
Carbs: 8g
Fat: 12g
Protein: 22g

83. Cheese & Ham Stuffed Turkey Breast

Preparation time: 15 minutes
Cooking time: 30 minutes
Servings: 4

Ingredients:
1 lb. turkey breast
2 ham slices
2 cheddar cheese slices
½ cup breadcrumbs
½ tsp garlic powder
½ tsp thyme
½ tsp tarragon
1 egg, beaten
Salt and black pepper to taste

Directions:
Preheat the air fryer oven to 350 F. Butterfly the turkey breast and place it between 2 plastic wraps. Flatten with a rolling pin to the ¼-inch thickness and lay on a clean surface.
Season with salt, pepper, garlic powder, thyme, and tarragon. Top with cheddar and ham slices and roll up, securing the edges with toothpicks.
Dip the prepared cordon bleu in egg first, then coat with breadcrumbs. Press Start and cook for 30 minutes until golden brown. Serve warm.

Nutrition:
Calories: 140
Carbs: 0g
Fat: 3g
Protein: 0g

84. Pineapple Chicken Kabobs with Sesame Seeds

Preparation time: 15 minutes
Cooking time: 14 minutes
Servings: 4

Ingredients:
1 lb. chicken tenders
½ cup of soy sauce
½ cup pineapple juice
¼ cup sesame oil
2 cloves garlic, chopped
1 tbsp fresh ginger, grated
4 scallions, chopped
2 tbsp toasted sesame seeds

Directions:
Preheat your air fryer oven on "Air Fry" function to 390 F. Thread the chicken pieces onto the skewers and trim any fat.
Mix all the remaining fixing in a bowl.
Dip in the skewered chicken and place it in the cooking basket. Press Start and cook for12-14 minutes. Serve.

Nutrition:
Calories: 230
Carbs: 22g
Fat: 4g
Protein: 26g

85. Cayenne Turkey Breasts

Preparation time: 15 minutes
Cooking time: 15 minutes
Servings: 4

Ingredients:
1 lb. turkey breast, boneless and skinless
2 cups panko breadcrumbs
Cayenne pepper and salt to taste
1 stick butter, melted

Directions
Preheat on "Air Fry" function to 350 F. In a bowl, mix breadcrumbs, cayenne pepper, and salt. Brush the butter onto the turkey and coat with the breadcrumbs. Cook for 15 minutes.

Nutrition:
Calories: 105
Carbs: 0g
Fat: 1g
Protein: 24g

86. Herby Turkey Balls

Preparation time: 15 minutes
Cooking time: 15 minutes
Servings: 2

Ingredients:
Ingredients
½ lb. ground turkey
1 egg, beaten
1 cup breadcrumbs
1 tbsp dried thyme
½ tbsp dried parsley
Salt and black pepper to taste

Directions:

Preheat on "Air Fry" function to 350 F. In a bowl, place ground turkey, thyme, parsley, salt, and pepper. Mix, then shape the mixture into balls.
Dip in breadcrumbs, then in the egg, and finally in the breadcrumbs again. Place the nuggets in the basket and cook for 15 minutes.

Nutrition:
Calories: 370
Carbs: 43g
Fat: 13g
Protein: 20g

87. Mayo Chicken Breasts with Basil & Cheese

Preparation time: 15 minutes
Cooking time: 15 minutes
Servings: 4

Ingredients:
4 chicken breasts, cubed
1 tsp garlic powder
1 cup mayonnaise
Salt and black pepper to taste
½ cup cream cheese softened
Chopped basil for garnish

Directions:
In a bowl, mix cream cheese, mayonnaise, garlic powder, and salt. Add in the chicken and toss to coat. Place the chicken in the basket and Press Start. Cook for 15 minutes at 380 F on "Air Fry" function. Serve garnished with roughly chopped fresh basil.

Nutrition:
Calories: 165
Carbs: 4g
Fat: 3g
Protein: 28g

88. Tangy Chicken Drumsticks with Cauliflower

Preparation time: 15 minutes
Cooking time: 20 minutes
Servings: 4

Ingredients:
1 lb. chicken drumsticks
½ tsp oregano
¼ cup oats
¼ cup milk
1 cup cauliflower florets, steamed
1 egg
1 tbsp cayenne pepper powder
Salt and black pepper to taste

Directions:
Preheat on "Air Fry" function to 350 F. Season the drumsticks with salt and pepper and rub them with the milk. Put all the other fixing, except for the egg, in a food processor.
Process until smooth. Dip each drumstick in the egg first, and then in the oat mixture. Arrange it on a greased baking tray. Press Start and cook in the oven for 20 minutes. Serve warm.

Nutrition:
Calories: 162
Carbs: 3g
Fat: 4g
Protein: 26g

89. Hot Curried Chicken Wings

Preparation time: 2 hours
Cooking time: 14 minutes
Servings: 2

Ingredients:
8 chicken wings
1 tbsp water
4 tbsp potato starch
2 tbsp hot curry paste
½ tbsp baking powder

Directions
In a bowl, combine curry paste with 1 tbsp of water. Put in the wings, then toss to coat. Cover the bowl with cling plastic, then refrigerate for 2 hours. Preheat on "Air Fry" function to 370 degrees. In a bowl, mix baking powder and potato starch. Dip in the wings. Transfer to a lined baking dish, press Start, and cook for 14 minutes.

Nutrition:
Calories: 252
Carbs: 50g
Fat: 3g
Protein: 11g

90. Red Thai Turkey Drumsticks in Coconut Milk

Preparation time: 25 minutes
Cooking time: 23 minutes
Servings: 2

Ingredients:
1 tablespoon red curry paste
1/2 teaspoon cayenne pepper
1 ½ tablespoons minced ginger
2 turkey drumsticks
1/4 cup coconut milk
1 teaspoon kosher salt
1/3 teaspoon ground pepper, to more to taste

Directions:
Put turkey drumsticks with all the fixing, let it marinate overnight.
Cook turkey drumsticks at 380 degrees f for 23 minutes; make sure to flip them over at half-time.
Serve with the salad on the side.

Nutrition:
Calories 298
Fat 16.3g
Carbs 5.3g
Protein 32.3g
Sugars 1.5g
Fiber 2.6g

91. Fried Turkey with Lemon and Herbs

Preparation time: 45 minutes
Cooking time: 28 minutes
Servings: 6

Ingredients:
1 ½ tablespoon yellow mustard
1 ½ tablespoons herb seasoning blend
1/3 cup tamari sauce
1 ½ tablespoon olive oil
1/2 lemon, juiced
3 turkey drumsticks
1/3 cup pear or apple cider vinegar

2 sprigs rosemary, chopped

Directions:

Dump all ingredients into a mixing dish. Let it marinate overnight.

Set your air fryer to cook at 355 degrees f.

Season turkey drumsticks with salt and black pepper and roast them at 355 degrees f for 28 minutes—Cook one drumstick at a time.

Pause the machine after 14 minutes and flip turkey drumstick.

Nutrition:

Calories 244
Fat 16g
Carbs 8g
Protein 11g
Sugars 3.9g
Fiber 0.7g

92. Chicken Sausage with Nestled Eggs

Preparation time: 20 minutes
Cooking time: 17 minutes
Servings: 6

Ingredients:

6 eggs
2 bell peppers, seeded and sliced
1 teaspoon dried oregano
1 teaspoon hot paprika
1 teaspoon freshly cracked black pepper
6 chicken sausages
1 teaspoon of sea salt
1 1/2 shallots, cut into wedges
1 teaspoon dried basil

Directions:

Take four ramekins and divide chicken sausages, shallot, and bell pepper among those ramekins. Cook at 315 degrees f for about 12 minutes.

Now, crack an egg into each ramekin. Sprinkle the eggs with hot paprika, basil, oregano, salt, and cracked black pepper—Cook for 5 more minutes at 405 degrees f.

Nutrition:

Calories 211
Fat 14.6g
Carbs 5.9g
Protein 14.7g
Sugars 1.4g
Fiber 0.7g

93. Parmesan Chicken Nuggets

Preparation time: 10 minutes
Cooking time: 8 minutes
Servings: 4

Ingredients:

1-pound chicken breast, ground
1 teaspoon hot paprika
2 teaspoon sage, ground
1/3 teaspoon powdered ginger
1/2 teaspoon dried thyme
1/3 teaspoon ground black pepper, to taste
1 teaspoon kosher salt
2 tablespoons melted butter
3 eggs, beaten
1/2 cup parmesan cheese, grated

Directions:

In a mixing bowl, thoroughly combine ground chicken with spices and an egg. After that, stir in the melted butter; mix to combine well.

Mix the remaining eggs in a shallow bowl.

Form the mixture into chicken nugget shapes; now, coat them with the beaten eggs; then, dredge them in the grated parmesan cheese.

Cook in the preheated air fryer at 405 degrees f for 8 minutes.

Nutrition:

Calories 347
Fat 23.6g
Carbs 1.5g
Protein 30.5g
Sugars 0.5g
Fiber 0g

94. Tangy and Buttery Chicken

Preparation time: 20 minutes
Cooking time: 13 minutes
Servings: 4
Ingredient:

½ tablespoon Worcestershire sauce
1 teaspoon finely grated orange zest
2 tablespoons melted butter
½ teaspoon smoked paprika
4 chicken drumsticks, rinsed and halved
1 teaspoon sea salt flakes
1 tablespoon cider vinegar
1/2 teaspoon mixed peppercorns, freshly cracked

Directions:

Firstly, pat the chicken drumsticks dry. Coat them with the melted butter on all sides. Toss the chicken drumsticks with the other ingredients.

Transfer them to the air fryer cooking basket and roast for about 13 minutes at 345 degrees f.

Nutrition:

Calories 264
Fat 18.6g
Carbs 0.9g
Protein 23.6g
Sugars 0.4g
Fiber 0.1g

95. Easy Turkey Kabobs

Preparation time: 15 minutes
Cooking time: 10 minutes
Servings: 8

Ingredients:

1 cup parmesan cheese, grated
1 ½ cups of water
14 ounces ground turkey
2 small eggs, beaten
1 teaspoon ground ginger
2 ½ tablespoons vegetable oil
1 cup chopped fresh parsley
2 tablespoons almond meal
3/4 teaspoon salt
1 heaping teaspoon fresh rosemary, finely chopped
1/2 teaspoon ground allspice

Directions:

Combine all of the fixings in a bowl. Knead the mixture with your hands.

Then, take small portions and gently roll them into balls.
Now, preheat your air fryer to 380 degrees f. Air fry for 8 to 10 minutes in the air fryer basket. Serve on a serving platter with skewers and eat with your favorite dipping sauce.
Nutrition:
Calories 360
Fat 31g
Carbs 3.9g
Protein 14.2g
Sugars 0.2g
Fiber 0.6g

96. Turkey Breasts with Greek Mustard Sauce

Preparation time: 1 hour & 13 minutes
Cooking time: 18 minutes
Servings: 4
Ingredients:
1/2 teaspoon cumin powder
2 pounds turkey breasts, quartered
2 cloves garlic, smashed
½ teaspoon hot paprika
2 tablespoons melted butter
1 teaspoon fine sea salt
Freshly cracked mixed peppercorns, to savor
Fresh juice of 1 lemon
For the mustard sauce:
1 ½ tablespoons mayonnaise
1 ½ cups Greek yogurt
1/2 tablespoon yellow mustard
Directions:
Grab a medium-sized mixing dish and combine the garlic and melted butter; rub this mixture evenly over the turkey's surface.
Add the cumin powder, followed by paprika, salt, peppercorns, and lemon juice—place in your refrigerator at least 55 minutes.
Set the air fryer to cook at 375 degrees f. Roast the turkey for 18 minutes, turning halfway through; roast in batches.
In the meantime, make the mustard sauce by mixing all ingredients for the sauce. Serve warm roasted turkey with the mustard sauce.
Nutrition:
Calories 471
Fat 23.6g
Carbs 4.1g
Protein 56g
Sugars 2.4g
Fiber 0.3g

97. Country-Style Nutty Turkey Breast

Preparation time: 30 minutes
Cooking time: 25 minutes
Servings: 2
Ingredients:
1 ½ tablespoons coconut aminos
1/2 tablespoon xanthan gum
2 bay leaves
1/3 cup dry sherry
1 ½ tablespoons chopped walnuts
1 teaspoon shallot powder
1-pound turkey breasts, sliced
1 teaspoon garlic powder
2 teaspoons olive oil
1/2 teaspoon onion salt
1/2 teaspoon red pepper flakes, crushed
1 teaspoon ground black pepper
Directions:
Begin by preheating your air fryer to 395 degrees f.
Place all ingredients, minus chopped walnuts, in a mixing bowl. Let it marinate at least 1 hour.
After that, cook the marinated turkey breast for approximately 23 minutes or until heated through.
Pause the machine, scatter chopped walnuts over the top and air-fry an additional 5 minutes.
Nutrition:
Calories 395
Fat 19.5g
Carbs 1.1g
Protein 51.5g
Sugars 0.4g
Fiber 0.5g

98. Eggs and Sausage with Keto Rolls

Preparation time: 40 minutes
Cooking time:
14 minutes
Servings: 6
Ingredients:
1 teaspoon dried dill weed
1 teaspoon mustard seeds
6 turkey sausages
3 bell peppers, seeded and thinly sliced
6 medium-sized eggs
1/2 teaspoon fennel seeds
1 teaspoon of sea salt
1/3 teaspoon freshly cracked pink peppercorns
Keto rolls:
1/2 cup ricotta cheese, crumbled
1 cup part-skim mozzarella cheese, shredded
1 egg
1/2 cup coconut flour
1/2 cup almond flour
1 teaspoon baking soda
2 tablespoons plain whey protein isolate
Directions:
Set your air fryer to cook at 325 degrees f. Cook the sausages and bell peppers in the air fryer cooking basket for 8 minutes.
Crack the eggs into the ramekins; sprinkle them with salt, dill weed, mustard seeds, fennel seeds, and cracked peppercorns—Cook an additional 12 minutes at 395 degrees f.
For the keto rolls, microwave the cheese for 1 minute 30 seconds, stirring twice. Add the cheese to the bowl of a food processor and blend well. Fold in the egg and mix again.
Add in the flour, baking soda, and plain whey protein isolate; blend again. Scrape the batter onto the center of a lightly greased cling film.
Form the dough into a disk and transfer to your freezer to cool; cut into 6 pieces and transfer to a parchment-lined baking pan (make sure to grease your hands.

Bake in the preheated air fryer oven at 400 degrees f for about 14 minutes.
Serve eggs and sausages on keto rolls.

Nutrition:

Calories 494
Fat 30.1g
Carbs 9.2g
Protein 45.1g
Sugars 2.3g
Fiber 2.1g

99. Bacon-Wrapped Turkey with Cheese

Preparation time: 20 minutes
Cooking time: 13 minutes
Servings: 2

Ingredients:

1 ½ small-sized turkey breast, chop into 12 pieces
12 thin slices asiago cheese
Paprika, to taste
sea salt
ground black pepper
12 rashers bacon

Directions:

Layout the bacon rashers; place 1 slice of asiago cheese on each bacon piece.
Top with turkey, season with paprika, salt, and pepper, and roll them up; secure with a cocktail stick.
Set on "Air Fry" at 365 degrees f for 13 minutes.

Nutrition:

Calories 568
Fat 34.6g
Carbs 0.7g
Protein 59g
Sugars 0.6g
Fiber 0.1g

100. Italian-Style Spicy Chicken Breasts

Preparation time: 20 minutes
Cooking time: 11 minutes
Servings: 4

Ingredients:

2 ounces Asiago cheese, cut into sticks
1/3 cup tomato paste
1/2 teaspoon garlic paste
2 chicken breasts, cut in half lengthwise
1/2 cup green onions, chopped
1 tablespoon chili sauce
1/2 cup roasted vegetable stock
1 tablespoon sesame oil
1 teaspoon salt
2 teaspoons unsweetened cocoa
1/2 teaspoon sweet paprika, or more to taste

Directions:

Sprinkle chicken breasts with the salt and sweet paprika; drizzle with chili sauce. Now, place a stick of asiago cheese in the middle of each chicken breast.
Then, tie the whole thing using a kitchen string; give a drizzle of sesame oil.
Transfer the stuffed chicken to the cooking basket.
Put the other ingredients and toss to coat the chicken.
Afterward, cook for about 11 minutes at 395 degrees f. Serve the chicken on two serving plates, garnish with fresh or pickled salad and serve immediately.

Nutrition:

Calories 390
Fat 12.6g
Carbs 7.5g
Protein 54g
Sugars 4.5g
Fiber 1.7g

101. Classic Chicken Nuggets

Preparation time: 20 minutes
Cooking time: 10 minutes
Servings: 4

Ingredients:

1 ½ pounds chicken tenderloins, cut into small pieces
1/2 teaspoon garlic salt
1/2 teaspoon cayenne pepper
1/4 teaspoon black pepper, freshly cracked
4 tablespoons olive oil
2 scoops low-carb unflavored protein powder
4 tablespoons parmesan cheese, freshly grated

Directions:

Warm your air fryer to 390 degrees f.
Season each piece of the chicken with garlic salt, cayenne pepper, and black pepper.
In a mixing bowl, thoroughly combine the olive oil with protein powder and parmesan cheese. Dip each piece of chicken in the parmesan mixture.
Cook for 8 minutes, working in batches.
Afterward, if you want to warm the chicken nuggets, add them to the basket and cook for 1 minute more.

Nutrition:

Calories 327
Fat 17g
Carbs 1.3g
Protein 40g
Sugars 0.2g
Fiber 1g

102. Thai Chicken with Bacon

Preparation time: 50 minutes
Cooking time: 20 minutes
Servings: 4

Ingredients:

4 rashers smoked bacon
2 chicken fillets
1/2 teaspoon coarse sea salt
1/4 teaspoon black pepper, preferably freshly ground
1 teaspoon garlic, minced
1 (2-inch piece ginger, peeled and minced
1 teaspoon black mustard seeds
1 teaspoon mild curry powder
1/2 cup coconut milk
1/2 cup parmesan cheese, grated

Directions:

Warm your air fryer to 400 degrees f. Add the smoked bacon and cook in the preheated air fryer for 5 to 7 minutes. Reserve.
In a mixing bowl, place the chicken fillets, salt, black pepper, garlic, ginger, mustard seeds, curry powder, and milk. Let it marinate in your refrigerator for about 30 minutes.
In another bowl, place the grated parmesan cheese.
Dredge the chicken fillets through the parmesan mixture and transfer them to the cooking basket.

Reduce the temperature to 380 degrees f and cook the chicken for 6 minutes.
Turn them over and cook for a further 6 minutes.
Repeat the process until you have run out of ingredients. Serve with reserved bacon. Enjoy!

Nutrition:

Calories 612
Fat 44.1g
Carbs 8.6g
Protein 52g
Sugars 2.5g
Fiber 2.1g

103. Thanksgiving Turkey with Mustard Gravy

Preparation time: 50 minutes
Cooking time: 45 minutes
Servings: 6

Ingredients:

2 teaspoons butter, softened
1 teaspoon dried sage
2 sprigs rosemary, chopped
1 teaspoon salt
1/4 teaspoon ground black pepper
1 whole turkey breast
2 tablespoons turkey broth
2 tablespoons whole-grain mustard
1 tablespoon butter

Directions:

Warm your air fryer to 360 degrees f.
To make the rub, combine 2 tablespoons of butter, sage, rosemary, salt, and pepper; mix well to combine and spread it evenly over the turkey breast's surface.
Roast for 20 minutes in an air fryer cooking basket.
Flip the turkey breast over and cook for a further 15 to 16 minutes. Now, flip it back over and roast for 12 minutes more.
While the turkey is roasting, whisk the other ingredients in a saucepan. After that, spread the gravy all over the turkey breast.
Let the turkey rest for a few minutes before carving.

Nutrition:

Calories 384
Fat 8.2g
Carbs 2.5g
Protein 51.5g
Sugars 0.2g
Fiber 0.2g

104. Loaded Turkey Meatloaf with Cheese

Preparation time: 50 minutes
Cooking time: 45 minutes
Servings: 6

Ingredients:

2 pounds turkey mince
1/2 cup scallions, finely chopped
2 garlic cloves, finely minced
1 teaspoon dried thyme
1/2 teaspoon dried basil
3/4 cup Colby cheese, shredded
1 tablespoon tamari sauce
Salt and black pepper, to your liking
1/4 cup roasted red pepper tomato sauce
3/4 tablespoons olive oil
1 medium-sized egg, well beaten

Directions:

Sauté the turkey mince, scallions, garlic, thyme, and basil until just tender and fragrant in a preheated nonstick skillet over moderate heat.
Then set your air fryer to cook at 360 degrees.
Combine sautéed mixture with the cheese and tamari sauce, then form the mixture into a loaf shape.
Mix the remaining items and pour them over the meatloaf—Cook in the air fryer baking pan for 45 to 47 minutes. Eat warm.

Nutrition:

Calories 324
Fat 19.3g
Carbs 2.7g
Protein 35.5g
Sugars 1.1g
Fiber 0.6g

105. Buffalo Chicken Tenders

Preparation time: 60 minutes
Cooking time: 25 minutes
Servings: 5

Ingredients:

Nonstick cooking spray
2/3 cup panko breadcrumbs
½ tsp cayenne pepper
½ tsp paprika
½ tsp garlic powder
½ tsp salt
3 chicken breasts, boneless, skinless & cut into 10 strips
½ cup butter, melted
½ cup hot sauce

Directions:

Line a baking sheet with foil and spray with cooking spray.
Mix bread crumbs and seasonings in a shallow dish.
Dip chicken in crumb mixture to coat all sides. Lay on prepared pan and refrigerate 1 hour.
In a small bowl, whisk butter and hot sauce.
Place the baking pan in position 2 of the oven. Lightly spray the fryer basket with cooking spray.
Dip each piece of chicken in the butter mixture and place it in the basket. Place the basket on the baking pan.
Set oven to air fry at 400°F for 25 minutes. Turn chicken over halfway through cooking time. Serve immediately.

Nutrition:

Calories 371
Fat 23g
Carbs 10g
Protein 31g
Sugar 1g
Fiber 1g
Sodium 733mg

106. Spicy Chicken Nuggets

Preparation time: 15 minutes
Cooking time: 10 minutes
Servings: 6

Ingredients:

Nonstick cooking spray

¼ cup mayonnaise
2 tbsp. sweet chili sauce
1 tbsp. honey
1 tbsp. + 2 tsp hot sauce, divided
1 cup buttermilk
¾ cup flour
½ cup cornstarch
1 egg
½ tsp salt
¼ tsp pepper
1 cup panko bread crumbs
1 lb. chicken breasts, boneless, skinless & cut into 1-inch pieces

Directions:

Place the baking pan in position 2 of your air fryer oven. Grease the fryer basket with cooking spray.
In a small bowl, whisk mayonnaise, chili sauce, honey, and 2 teaspoons hot sauce. Cover until ready to use.
In a large bowl, whisk buttermilk, flour, cornstarch, egg, remaining hot sauce, salt, and pepper.
Place bread crumbs in a shallow dish.
Dip the chicken into buttermilk mixture one at a time, then roll in bread crumbs to coat. Place in fryer basket in a single layer; these will need to be cooked in batches. Lightly spray the nuggets with cooking spray.
Place basket in the air fryer oven and air fry at 375°F for 10 minutes. Cook chicken until golden brown outside and no longer pink inside, turning over halfway through cooking time. Repeat with remaining chicken pieces.
Serve drizzled with reserved sauce.

Nutrition:

Calories 459
Fat 11g
Carbs 41g
Protein 24g
Sugar 7g
Fiber 2g
Sodium 615mg

107. Turkey Meatloaf

Preparation time: 15 minutes
Cooking time: 55 minutes
Servings: 4

Ingredients:

¼ cup + 2 tbsp. ketchup, divided
2 tsp Worcestershire sauce
1 tsp olive oil
½ onion, chopped fine
1 1/3 lbs. lean ground turkey
½ cup bread crumbs, seasoned
1 egg
1 tsp salt
1 tsp marjoram

Directions:

Place rack in position 1 of the oven.
In a small bowl, stir 2 tablespoons ketchup and Worcestershire sauce.
Heat oil in a small skillet over low heat. Add onion and cook until translucent, about 3-5 minutes. Remove from heat.
In a medium bowl, combine turkey, onion, bread crumbs, egg, salt, marjoram, and remaining ketchup.
Transfer mixture to an 8-inch loaf pan. Spread sauce over the top.
Set your air fryer oven to bake at 350°F for 60 minutes. After 5 minutes, place the turkey loaf in the oven and bake 55-60 minutes.
Remove and let it rest 5 minutes before slicing and serving.

Nutrition:

Calories 354
Fat 16g
Carbs 18g
Protein 32g
Sugar 6g
Fiber 1g
Sodium 1112mg

108. Lacquered Duck Breasts

Preparation time: 15 minutes
Cooking time: 15 minutes
Servings: 4

Ingredients:

2 Margret duck breasts
¾ tsp salt, divided
¼ tsp pepper
4 tbsp. honey
3 tbsp. balsamic vinegar
¼ tsp cinnamon

Directions:

Place the baking pan in position 1 of the oven.
With a sharp knife, score the duck's skin, don't cut through to the flesh. Sprinkle both sides with ½ teaspoon salt and pepper.
Heat a large skillet over med-high heat. Add the duck, skin side down, and cook 5-6 minutes, or until fat is rendered. Transfer duck, and keep warm.
Drain the fat from the skillet. Add honey and vinegar and deglaze the pan, stirring up the browned bits from the bottom. Simmer mixture 2-3 minutes until it starts to thicken. Stir in ¼ teaspoon salt and cinnamon.
Set the oven to convection bake at 375°F for 15 minutes.
Add the duck to the skillet and turn to coat with sauce. After the oven has preheated for 5 minutes, place the duck on the baking pan and pour a little sauce over the top.
Cook another 7-10 minutes, turning duck over and adding more sauce halfway through until duck reaches medium-rare. Slice and serve immediately.

Nutrition:

Calories 184
Fat 4g
Carbs 20g
Protein 17g
Sugar 19g
Fiber 0g
Sodium 487mg

109. Copycat Chicken Sandwich

Preparation time: 15 minutes
Cooking time: 15 minutes
Servings: 4

Ingredients:

2 chicken breasts, boneless & skinless

1 cup buttermilk
1 tbsp. + 2 tsp paprika, divided
1 tbsp. + 1 ½ tsp garlic powder, divided
2 tsp salt, divided
2 tsp pepper, divided
4 brioche buns
1 cup flour
½ cup of corn starch
1 tbsp. onion powder
1 tbsp. cayenne pepper
½ cup mayonnaise
1 tsp hot sauce
Sliced pickles

Directions:

Put the chicken between the two sheets of plastic wrap and pound to ½-inch thick. Cut crosswise to get 4 cutlets.
In a large bowl, whisk buttermilk and one teaspoon each paprika, garlic powder, salt, and pepper. Add the chicken, cover, and refrigerate overnight.
Place the buns on the baking pan and place it in position 2 of the oven. Set to toast for about 2-5 minutes depending on how toasted you want them. Set aside.
In a medium shallow dish, combine flour, cornstarch, onion powder, cayenne pepper, and remaining paprika, garlic powder, salt, and pepper.
Whisk in 2-3 tablespoons of the buttermilk batter chicken was marinating in until smooth.
Lightly spray fryer basket with cooking spray.
Dredge chicken in the flour mixture forming a thick coating of the batter—place in the fryer basket.
Place the basket in the oven. Set oven to air fryer at 375°F for 10 minutes. Cook until crispy and golden brown, turning chicken over halfway through cooking time.
In a small bowl, whisk mayonnaise, hot sauce, 1 teaspoon paprika, and ½ teaspoon garlic powder.
To serve, spread top of buns with mayonnaise mixture—place chicken on bottom buns and top with pickles then top bun.

Nutrition:

Calories 689
Fat 27g
Carbs 71g
Protein 38g
Sugar 7g
Fiber 4g
Sodium 1734mg

110. Mini Pot Pies

Preparation time: 15 minutes
Cooking time: 20 minutes
Servings: 16

Ingredients:

2 cans large flaky biscuits, refrigerated
6 oz. turkey, cooked & chopped fine
3 ½ cups turkey gravy
2 cups of mixed vegetables
1 cup cheddar cheese, grated

Directions:

Place the baking pan in position 1 of the oven. Spray 3 6-cup muffin tins with cooking spray.
Gently pull each biscuit until it is double in size. Press into prepared tins, pressing up the sides until the edge is at the top of the cup.
In a large bowl, stir turkey, gravy, and vegetables.
Spoon mixture into biscuits. Top with cheese.
Set oven to bake at 350°F for 25 minutes. After 5 minutes, place muffin tin, one at a time, in the oven. Bake until golden brown, about 20-22 minutes.
Repeat with remaining tins. Serve warm.

Nutrition:

Calories 324
Fat 8g
Carbs 24g
Protein 9g
Sugar 1g
Fiber 1g
Sodium 790mg

111. Popcorn Turkey

Preparation time: 15 minutes
Cooking time: 10 minutes
Servings: 4

Ingredients:

Nonstick cooking spray
1 cup flour
2 eggs
½ cup milk
2 tbsp. Cajun seasoning
2 cups bread crumbs
1 large turkey breast, cut into 1-inch pieces

Directions:

Place the baking pan in position 2 of the oven. Lightly grease the fryer basket with cooking spray.
In a large bowl, whisk flour, eggs, milk, and seasoning.
Place bread crumbs in a shallow dish.
Add the turkey to the batter and stir to coat. Roll each turkey piece in the bread crumbs and place them in the fryer basket; these may need to be cooked in batches. Spray them lightly with cooking spray.
Set to air fry at 375°F for 10 minutes. Cook turkey nuggets until crisp and golden brown, turning over halfway through cooking time. Serve with your favorite dipping sauce.

Nutrition:

Calories 655
Fat 11g
Carbs 64g
Protein 78g
Sugar 5g
Fiber 3g
Sodium 690mg
Potassium 855mg

112. Italian Chicken Casserole

Preparation time: 15 minutes
Cooking time: 30 minutes
Servings: 4

Ingredients:

Nonstick cooking spray.
2 tbsp. olive oil
1 cup chicken breasts, boneless, skinless & cut in 1-inch pieces
2/3 onion, chopped
1 clove garlic, chopped fine

1 cup elbow macaroni, cook according to pkg. directions, drain
14 ½ oz. tomatoes, diced
1 ¼ cups mozzarella cheese, grated
¼ cup fresh parsley, chopped
½ tsp salt
¼ tsp pepper
¼ cup bread crumbs
1/3 cup parmesan cheese, grated
2 tbsp. butter, melted

Directions:

Place the rack in position 1 of the oven. Spray an 8-inch square baking dish with cooking spray.
Heat oil in a medium skillet over medium heat. Add chicken and cook 3 minutes, stirring occasionally.
Add the onions and garlic and cook until onions are soft and chicken is no longer pink about 5 minutes.
Mix pasta and chicken in a large bowl. Stir in tomatoes with their juice, mozzarella cheese, parsley, salt, and pepper. Transfer to prepared baking dish.
Set oven to bake at 400°F for 35 minutes.
In a small bowl, stir bread crumbs, parmesan cheese, and butter. Sprinkle on top of casserole.
Once the oven has preheated for 5 minutes, add casserole and bake 30 minutes until the top is golden brown. Serve.

Nutrition:

Calories 427
Fat 17g
Carbs 36g
Protein 30g
Sugar 7g
Fiber 4g
Sodium 1011mg

113. Roast Duck

Preparation time: 15 minutes
Cooking time: 1 hour
Servings: 6

Ingredients:

6 **Ingredients:**
3 lb. duck
1 tsp salt
3 tbsp. crushed red pepper flakes
3 tbsp. soy sauce, divided
3 tbsp. honey
2 tbsp. rice vinegar

Directions:

Place the duck in an 8x11-inch baking dish.
Stir the salt and pepper flakes in a small bowl, then rub over the duck's skin. Sprinkle 2 tablespoons soy sauce over duck. Cover and refrigerate 2 hours.
Place rack in position 1 and set the oven to convection bake at 375°F for 5 minutes.
In a small bowl, whisk honey, vinegar, and remaining soy sauce. Brush over the duck.
Once the oven has preheated, place duck inside and cook 1 hour. Serve.

Nutrition:

Calories 519
Fat 35g
Carbs 11g
Protein 40g
Sugar 9g
Fiber 1g
Sodium 772mg

114. Sweet & Spicy Chicken

Preparation time: 15 minutes
Cooking time: 30 minutes
Servings: 6

Ingredients:

6 chicken breasts, skinless, boneless, cut in 1-inch pieces
1 cup of corn starch
2 cups of water
1 cup ketchup
½ cup brown sugar
1 tbsp. sesame oil
3 tbsp. soy sauce
2 tbsp. black sesame seeds
2 tbsp. white sesame seeds
½ tsp red pepper flakes
½ tsp garlic powder
2 tbsp. green onion, chopped

Directions:

Place the baking pan in position 2. Lightly spray fryer basket with cooking spray.
Place the cornstarch in a large bowl. Put the chicken and toss to coat the chicken thoroughly.
Work it in batches, place chicken in a single layer in the basket, and place on baking pan. Set oven to air fryer at 350°F for 10 minutes. Stir the chicken halfway through cooking time—transfer chicken to the baking sheet.
Mix the remaining ingredients, except green onion, in a large skillet over medium heat. Bring to a boil, stirring occasionally—Cook within about 3-5 minutes.
Add chicken and stir to coat. Cook another 3-5 minutes, stirring frequently. Serve garnished with green onions.

Nutrition:

Calories 556
Fat 12g
Carbs 50g
Protein 62g
Sugar 26g
Fiber 1g
Sodium 730mg

115. Guacamole Stuffed Chicken

Preparation time: 15 minutes
Cooking time: 10 minutes
Servings: 4

Ingredients:

Nonstick cooking spray
2 chicken breasts, boneless & skinless
½ cup guacamole
2/3 cup cheddar cheese, grated
1 cup panko bread crumbs
½ tsp Adobo seasoning

Directions:

Place the baking pan in position 2. Spray the fryer basket with cooking spray.
Cut the chicken breasts in half, similar to butterflying them but cut all the way through. Place the chicken

between two sheets of plastic wrap and pound really thin.

Spread 2 tablespoons guacamole over each piece of chicken. Sprinkle with the cheese. Fold the chicken pieces in half, covering the filling.

Mix the bread crumbs plus seasoning in a shallow dish. Coat each side of chicken with mixture and place in the fryer basket.

Place the basket in the air fryer oven and set to air fry at 375°F for 10 minutes. Turn chicken over halfway through cooking time. Serve immediately.

Nutrition:

Calories 363
Fat 15g
Carbs 22g
Protein 35g
Sugar 2g
Fiber 3g
Sodium 441mg

116. Buttermilk Marinated Chicken

Preparation Time: 10 minutes
Cooking Time: 25 minutes
Servings: 6

Ingredients:

3-lb. whole chicken
1 tablespoon salt
1-pint buttermilk

Directions:

Place the whole chicken in a large bowl and drizzle salt on top.

Pour the buttermilk over it and leave the chicken soaked overnight.

Cover the chicken bowl and refrigerate overnight.

Remove the chicken and fix it on the rotisserie rod in the air fryer.

Air Roast, and set the cooking time to 25 minutes. Set the temperature at 370 degrees F.

Close its lid and allow the chicken to roast.

Serve warm.

Nutrition:

Calories 284
Fat 7.9 g
Carbs 46 g
Fiber 3.6 g
Sugar 5.5 g
Protein 17.9 g

117. Thyme Turkey Breast

Preparation Time: 10 minutes
Cooking Time: 40 minutes
Servings: 4

Ingredients:

2 lb. turkey breast
Salt, to taste
Black pepper, to taste
4 tablespoon butter, melted
3 cloves garlic, minced
1 teaspoon thyme, chopped
1 teaspoon rosemary, chopped

Directions:

Mix butter with salt, black pepper, garlic, thyme, and rosemary in a bowl.

Rub this seasoning over the turkey breast liberally and place in the Air Fryer basket.

Set cook to 40 minutes on Air Fry. Set the temperature at 375 degrees F.

Once preheated, place the Air fryer basket inside the oven.

Slice and serve fresh.

Nutrition:

Calories 334
Fat 4.7 g
Sodium 1 mg
Carbs 54.1 g
Fiber 7 g
Sugar 3.3 g
Protein 26.2 g

118. Roasted Duck

Preparation Time: 10 minutes
Cooking Time: 3 hours
Servings: 12

Ingredients:

6 lb. whole Pekin duck
salt
5 garlic cloves chopped
1 lemon, chopped
Glaze
1/2 cup balsamic vinegar
1 lemon, juiced
1/4 cup honey

Directions:

Place the Pekin duck in a baking tray and add garlic, lemon, and salt on top.

Whisk honey, vinegar, and honey in a bowl. Brush this glaze over the duck liberally.

Marinate overnight in the refrigerator.

Remove the duck from the marinade and fix it on the rotisserie rod in the air fryer oven.

Select Air Roast, then set the cooking time to 3 hours at 350 degrees F.

Close its lid and allow the duck to roast. Serve warm.

Nutrition:

Calories 387
Fat 6 g
Sodium 154 mg
Carbs 37.4 g
Fiber 2.9 g
Sugar 15.3 g
Protein 14.6 g

119. Chicken Drumsticks

Preparation Time: 10 minutes
Cooking Time: 20 minutes
Servings: 8

Ingredients:

8 chicken drumsticks
2 tablespoon olive oil
1 teaspoon salt
1 teaspoon pepper
1 teaspoon garlic powder
1 teaspoon paprika
1/2 teaspoon cumin

Directions:

Mix olive oil with salt, black pepper, garlic powder, paprika, and cumin in a bowl.

Rub this mixture liberally over all the drumsticks.
Place these drumsticks in the air fryer basket.
Set the cooking time to 20 minutes at 375 degrees F.
Flip the drumsticks when cooked halfway through.
Resume air frying for another rest of the 10 minutes.
Serve warm.

Nutrition:

Calories 212
Fat 11.8 g
Sodium 321 mg
Carbs 14.6 g
Fiber 4.4 g
Sugar 8 g
Protein 17.3 g

120. Blackened Chicken Bake

Preparation Time: 10 minutes
Cooking Time: 18 minutes
Servings: 4

Ingredients:

4 chicken breasts
2 teaspoon olive oil
Seasoning:
1 1/2 tablespoon brown sugar
1 teaspoon paprika
1 teaspoon dried oregano
1/4 teaspoon garlic powder
1/2 teaspoon salt and pepper
Garnish:
Chopped parsley

Directions:

Mix olive oil with brown sugar, paprika, oregano, garlic powder, salt, and black pepper in a bowl.
Place the chicken breasts in the baking tray of the air fry oven.
Pour and rub this mixture liberally over all the chicken breasts.
Choose "Bake" set the cooking time to 18 minutes at 425 degrees F. Once done, serve warm.

Nutrition:

Calories 412
Fat 24.8 g
Sodium 132 mg
Carbs 43.8 g
Fiber 3.9 g
Sugar 2.5 g
Protein 18.9 g

121. Crusted Chicken Drumsticks

Preparation Time: 10 minutes
Cooking Time: 10 minutes
Servings: 4

Ingredients:

1 lb. chicken drumsticks
1/2 cup buttermilk
1/2 cup panko breadcrumbs
1/2 cup flour
1/4 teaspoon baking powder
Spice Mixture:
1/2 teaspoon salt
1/2 teaspoon celery salt
1/4 teaspoon oregano
1/4 teaspoon cayenne
1 teaspoon paprika
1/4 teaspoon garlic powder
1/4 teaspoon dried thyme
1/2 teaspoon ground ginger
1/2 teaspoon white pepper
1/2 teaspoon black pepper
3 tablespoon butter melted

Directions:

Soak chicken in the buttermilk and cover to marinate overnight in the refrigerator.
Mix spices with flour, breadcrumbs, and baking powder in a shallow tray.
Remove the chicken from the milk and coat them well with the flour spice mixture
Place the chicken drumsticks in the air fryer basket.
Pour the melted butter over the drumsticks
Air Fry, then set the cooking time to 10 minutes. Set the temperature at 425 degrees F.
Flip the drumsticks and resume cooking for another 10 minutes. Serve warm.

Nutrition:

Calories 331
Fat 2.5 g
Sodium 595 mg
Carbs 69 g
Fiber 12.2 g
Sugar 12.5 g
Protein 28.7g

122. Roasted Turkey Breast

Preparation Time: 10 minutes
Cooking Time: 50 minutes
Servings: 6

Ingredients:

3 lb. boneless turkey breast
¼ cup mayonnaise
2 teaspoon poultry seasoning
1 teaspoon salt
½ teaspoon garlic powder
¼ teaspoon black pepper

Directions:

Whisk all the ingredients, including turkey, in a bowl, and coat it well.
Place the boneless turkey breast in the air fryer basket.
Rotate the dial to select the "Air fry" mode.
Set the cooking time to 50 minutes at 350 degrees F.
Once preheated, place the air fryer basket in the oven and close its lid to bake.
Slice and serve.

Nutrition:

Calories 322
Fat 11.8 g
Sodium 321 mg
Carbs 14.6 g
Fiber 4.4 g
Sugar 8 g
Protein 17.3 g

123. Brine Soaked Turkey

Preparation Time: 10 minutes
Cooking Time: 45 minutes
Servings: 8

Ingredients:

7 lb. bone-in, skin-on turkey breast

Brine:
1/2 cup salt
1 lemon
1/2 onion
3 cloves garlic, smashed
5 sprigs fresh thyme
3 bay leaves
black pepper
Turkey Breast:
4 tablespoon butter, softened
1/2 teaspoon black pepper
1/2 teaspoon garlic powder
1/4 teaspoon dried thyme
1/4 teaspoon dried oregano
Directions:
Mix the turkey brine ingredients in a pot and soak the turkey in the brine overnight.
The following day, remove the soaked turkey from the brine.
Whisk the butter, black pepper, garlic powder, oregano, and thyme.
Brush the butter mixture over the turkey, then place it in a baking tray.
Air Roast within 45 minutes, then set the temperature at 370 degrees F.
Once preheated, place the turkey baking tray in the oven and close its lid.
Slice and serve warm.
Nutrition:
Calories 397
Fat 15.4 g
Sodium 203 mg
Carbs 58.5 g
Sugar 1.1 g
Fiber 4 g
Protein 7.9 g

124. Turkey Meatballs

Preparation Time: 10 minutes
Cooking Time: 20 minutes
Servings: 6
Ingredients:
1.5 lb. turkey mince
1 red bell pepper, deseeded and chopped
1 large egg, beaten
4 tablespoons parsley, minced
1 tablespoon cilantro, minced
Salt, to taste
Black pepper, to taste
Directions:
Toss all the meatball ingredients in a bowl and mix well.
Make small meatballs out this mixture and place them in the air fryer basket.
Set the cooking time to 20 minutes, Air Fry. Set the temperature at 375 degrees F.
Once preheated, place the air fryer basket inside and close its lid. Serve warm.
Nutrition:
Calories 338
Fat 9.7 g
Sodium 245 mg
Carbs 32.5 g
Fiber 0.3 g
Sugar 1.8 g
Protein 10.3 g

125. Lemon Pepper Turkey

Preparation Time: 10 minutes
Cooking Time: 45 minutes
Servings: 6
Ingredients:
3 lbs. turkey breast
2 tablespoons oil
1 tablespoon Worcestershire sauce
1 teaspoon lemon pepper
1/2 teaspoon salt
Directions:
Whisk everything in a bowl and coat the turkey liberally.
Place the turkey in the air fryer basket. Set the cooking time to 45 minutes.
Set the temperature at 375 degrees F. Serve warm.
Nutrition:
Calories 391
Fat 2.8 g
Sodium 62 mg
Carbs 36.5 g
Fiber 9.2 g
Sugar 4.5 g
Protein 6.6

126. Ground Chicken Meatballs

Preparation Time: 10 minutes
Cooking Time: 10 minutes
Servings: 4
Ingredients:
1-lb. ground chicken
1/3 cup panko
1 teaspoon salt
2 teaspoons chives
1/2 teaspoon garlic powder
1 teaspoon thyme
1 egg
Directions:
Toss all the meatball ingredients in a bowl and mix well.
Make small meatballs out this mixture and place them in the air fryer basket.
Air Fry within 10 minutes at 350 degrees F. Serve warm.
Nutrition:
Calories 453
Fat 2.4 g
Sodium 216 mg
Carbs 18 g
Fiber 2.3 g
Sugar 1.2 g
Protein 23.2 g

127. Parmesan Chicken Meatballs

Preparation Time: 10 minutes
Cooking Time: 12 minutes
Servings: 4
Ingredients:
1-lb. ground chicken
1 large egg, beaten
½ cup Parmesan cheese, grated

½ cup pork rinds, ground
1 teaspoon garlic powder
1 teaspoon paprika
1 teaspoon kosher salt
½ teaspoon pepper
Crust:
½ cup pork rinds, ground

Directions:

Toss all the meatball ingredients in a bowl and mix well.
Make small meatballs out this mixture and roll them in the pork rinds.
Place the coated meatballs in the air fryer basket.
Select Bake mode, set the cooking time to 12 minutes at 400 degrees F.
Once preheated, place the air fryer basket inside and close its lid. Serve warm.

Nutrition:

Calories 529
Fat 17 g
Sodium 391 mg
Carbs 55 g
Fiber 6 g
Sugar 8 g
Protein 41g

128. Easy Italian Meatballs

Preparation Time: 10 minutes
Cooking Time: 13 minutes
Servings: 4

Ingredients:

2-lb. lean ground turkey
¼ cup onion, minced
2 cloves garlic, minced
2 tablespoons parsley, chopped
2 eggs
1½ cup parmesan cheese, grated
½ teaspoon red pepper flakes
½ teaspoon Italian seasoning
Salt and black pepper to taste

Directions:

Toss all the meatball ingredients in a bowl and mix well.
Make small meatballs out this mixture and place them in the air fryer basket.
Air Fry within 13 minutes at 350 degrees F.
Flip the meatballs when cooked halfway through.
Serve warm.

Nutrition:

Calories 472
Fat 25.8 g
Sodium 503 mg
Carbs 1.7 g
Fiber 0.3 g
Sugar 0.6 g
Protein 59.6 g

129. Oregano Chicken Breast

Preparation Time: 10 minutes
Cooking Time: 25 minutes
Servings: 6

Ingredients:

2 lbs. chicken breasts, minced
1 tablespoon avocado oil
1 teaspoon smoked paprika
1 teaspoon garlic powder
1 teaspoon oregano
1/2 teaspoon salt
Black pepper, to taste

Directions:

Toss all the meatball ingredients in a bowl and mix well.
Make small meatballs out this mixture and place them in the air fryer basket.
Air Fry within 25 minutes at 375 degrees F. Serve warm.

Nutrition:

Calories 352
Fat 14 g
Sodium 220 mg
Carbs 15.8 g
Fiber 0.2 g
Sugar 1 g
Protein 26 g

130. Lemon Chicken Breasts

Preparation Time: 10 minutes
Cooking Time: 30 minutes
Servings: 4

Ingredients:

1/4 cup olive oil
3 tablespoons garlic, minced
1/3 cup dry white wine
1 tablespoon lemon zest, grated
2 tablespoons lemon juice
1 1/2 teaspoons dried oregano, crushed
1 teaspoon thyme leaves, minced
Salt and black pepper
4 skin-on boneless chicken breasts
1 lemon, sliced

Directions:

Whisk everything in a baking pan to coat the chicken breasts well.
Place the lemon slices on top of the chicken breasts.
Spread the mustard mixture over the toasted bread slices.
Bake mode, and set the cooking time to 30 minutes at 370 degrees F.
Once preheated, place the baking pan inside and close its lid.
Serve warm.

Nutrition:

Calories 388
Fat 8 g
Sodium 339 mg
Carbs 8 g
Fiber 1 g
Sugar 2 g
Protein 13 g

Chapter 5. Meat Recipes

131. Simple Sirloin Roast

Preparation time: 15 minutes
Cooking time: 50 minutes
Servings: 8
Ingredients:
Sirloin roast – 2½ lb.
Salt and ground black pepper
Directions:
Rub the roast with salt and black pepper generously. Insert the rotisserie rod through the roast, one on each side of the rod.
Select "Roast" at 350 °F. Set the time for 50 minutes and press "Start."
When it's done, press the red lever to release the rod. Place the roast onto a platter for about 10 minutes before slicing. Cut the sirloin roast into desired-sized slices and serve.
Nutrition:
Calories 258
Carbs 0g
Fat 11.8g
Protein 37.9g

132. Herbed Chuck Roast

Preparation time: 15 minutes
Cooking time: 45 minutes
Servings: 5
Ingredients:
2 lbs. Beef chuck roast
1 tbsp Olive oil
1 tsp Dried rosemary, crushed
1 tsp dried thyme, crushed
Salt, as required
Directions:
In a bowl, add the oil, herbs, and salt and mix well. Coat the beef roast with herb mixture generously. Arrange the beef roast onto the greased cooking tray. Select "Air Fry" to 360 °F. Set the time for 45 minutes and press "Start."
Remove and place the roast onto a cutting board. With a piece of foil, cover the beef roast for about 20 minutes before slicing. With a sharp knife, cut the beef roast into desired-sized slices and serve.
Nutrition:
Calories 32
Carbs 0.3g
Fat 14.2g
Protein 55.1g

133. Seasoned Beef Top Roast

Preparation time: 15 minutes
Cooking time: 45 minutes
Servings: 5
Ingredients:
3 lb. Beef top roast
1 tbsp Olive oil
2 tbsp Montreal steak seasoning
Directions:
Coat the roast with oil and then rub with the seasoning generously. With kitchen twines, tie the roast to keep it compact. Arrange the roast onto the cooking tray.
Select "Air Fry" over 360 F. Set the time for 45 minutes
Remove and place the roast onto a platter for about 10 minutes before slicing. Slice into desired-sized slices and serve.
Nutrition:
Calories 269
Carbs 0g
Fat 9.9g
Protein 41.3g

134. Simple Beef Tenderloin

Preparation time: 15 minutes
Cooking time: 40 minutes
Servings: 4
Ingredients:
1 (3-lb.) Beef tenderloin, trimmed
2 tbsps. Olive oil
Salt and ground black pepper
Directions:
Rub tenderloin with oil and then season with salt and black pepper evenly. Arrange the tenderloin onto the greased cooking tray.
Select "Bake" and then adjust the temperature to 400 °F. Set the time for 40 minutes and press "Start."
Remove, then place the tenderloin onto a cutting board. With a piece of foil, cover the tenderloin for about 10 minutes before slicing. With a sharp knife, cut the tenderloin into desired-sized slices and serve.
Nutrition:
Calories 380
Carbs 0g
Fat 19.1g
Protein 49.2g

135. Strip Steak

Preparation time: 15 minutes
Cooking time: 8 minutes
Servings: 2
Ingredients:
9½-oz. New York strip steak
Salt and ground black pepper
1 tsp Olive oil
Directions:
Coat the steak with oil and then sprinkle with salt and black pepper evenly. Arrange the steak onto the greased cooking tray.
Arrange the pan in the bottom of the air fryer oven, then select "Air Fry" to 400 °F.
Set the time for 8 minutes and press "Start."
Remove, then place the steak onto a platter for about 10 minutes. Cut the steak into desired-sized slices and serve immediately.
Nutrition:
Calories 344
Carbs 0g
Fat 22.5g
Protein 36g

136. Bacon-Wrapped Filet Mignon

Preparation time: 15 minutes
Cooking time: 15 minutes

Servings: 2

Ingredients:

2 Bacon slices
2 Filet mignons
Salt and ground black pepper
Olive oil cooking spray

Directions:

Wrap 1 bacon slice around each filet mignon and secure with toothpicks. Season the fillets with the salt and black pepper lightly.

Arrange the filet mignon onto a rack and spray with cooking spray.

Select "Air Fry" to 375 °F. Set the time for 15 minutes and press "Start."

When it shows "Turn Food," turn the filets. Remove, then serve hot.

Nutrition:

Calories 360
Carbs 0.4g
Fat 19.6g
Protein 42.6g

137. Beef Jerky

Preparation time: 15 minutes
Cooking time: 3 hours
Servings: 4

Ingredients:

1½ lbs. Beef round, trimmed
½ cup Worcestershire sauce
½ cup Low-sodium soy sauce
2 tsp Honey
1 tsp Liquid smoke
2 tsp Onion powder
½ tsp Red pepper flakes, crushed
Ground black pepper

Directions:

In a zip-top bag, place the beef and freeze for 1-2 hours to firm up. Place the beef meat onto a cutting board and cut against the grain into 1/8-¼-inch strips.

In a large bowl, add the remaining ingredients and mix until thoroughly combined. Add the steak slices and coat with the mixture generously.

Refrigerate to marinate for about 4-6 hours. Remove the beef slices from the bowl and with paper towels; pat dries them.

Divide the steak strips onto the cooking trays and arrange them in an even layer.

Select "Dehydrate" and then adjust the temperature to 160 °F. Set the time for 3 hours and press "Start."

Once it shows "Add Food," insert 1 tray in the top position and another in the center position.

After 1½ hours, switch the position of cooking trays. Remove the trays, then serve.

Nutrition:

Calories 372
Carbs 12g
Fat 10.7g
Protein 53.8g

138. Meatballs

Preparation time: 15 minutes
Cooking time: 30 minutes
Servings: 8

Ingredients:

For Meatballs:
2 lb. Lean ground beef
2/3 cup Quick-cooking oats
½ cup Ritz crackers, crushed
1 can Evaporate milk
2 large eggs, beaten lightly
1 tsp Honey
1 tbsp Dried onion, minced
1 tsp Garlic powder
1 tsp ground cumin
Salt and ground black pepper
For Sauce:
1/3 cup Orange marmalade
1/3 cup Honey
1/3 cup Brown sugar
2 tbsp Cornstarch
2 tbsp Soy sauce
1-2 tbsp Hot sauce
1 tbsp Worcestershire sauce

Directions:

For meatballs: Add all the meatball ingredients into a bowl and mix until thoroughly combined. Make 1½-inch balls from the mixture.

Arrange half of the meatballs onto the greased cooking tray in a single layer.

Select "Air Fry" to 380 °F. Set the time for 15 minutes and press "Start."

When it shows "Turn Food," turn the meatballs. Remove, then repeat the process with the remaining meatballs.

Meanwhile, for the sauce: In a small pan, add all ingredients over medium heat and cook until thickened, stirring continuously. Serve the meatballs with the topping of sauce.

Nutrition:

Calories 411
Carbs 38.8g
Fat 11.1g
Protein 38.9g

139. Beef Burgers

Preparation time: 15 minutes
Cooking time: 18 minutes
Servings: 4

Ingredients:

For Burgers:
1 lb. Ground beef
½ cup Panko breadcrumbs
¼ cup Onion, chopped finely
3 tbsps. Dijon mustard
3 tsp Low-sodium soy sauce
2 tsp fresh rosemary, minced
Salt, as required
For Topping:
2 tbsp Dijon mustard
1 tbsp Brown sugar
1 tsp Soy sauce
4 Gruyere cheese slices

Directions:

Add all the burger ingredients into a bowl and mix until thoroughly combined. Make 4 equal-sized patties from the mixture. Arrange the patties onto the greased cooking tray.

Select "Air Fry" to 370 °F.
Set the time for 15 minutes and press "Start." When it shows "Add Food," insert the cooking rack in the center position. When it shows "Turn Food," turn the burgers.
Meanwhile, mix the mustard, brown sugar, and soy sauce in a small bowl to make the sauce. When done, remove and coat the burgers with the sauce.
Top each burger with 1 cheese slice. Return the tray and select "Broil." Set the time for 3 minutes and press "Start." Remove, and serve hot.

Nutrition:

Calories 402
Carbs 6.3g
Fat 18g
Protein 44.4g

140. Beef Casserole

Preparation time: 15 minutes
Cooking time: 25 minutes
Servings: 6

Ingredients:

2 lbs. Ground beef
2 tbsp taco seasoning
1 cup Cheddar cheese, shredded
1 cup Cottage cheese
1 cup of salsa

Directions:

In a bowl, add the beef and taco seasoning and mix well. Add the cheeses and salsa and stir to combine. Place the mixture into a baking dish that will fit in the Air Fryer Oven.
Choose "Air Fry" to 370 °F.
Set the time for 25 minutes and press "Start." After that, serve warm.

Nutrition:

Calories 412
Carbs 6.3g
Fat 16.5g
Protein 56.4g

141. Garlicky Pork Tenderloin

Preparation time: 15 minutes
Cooking time: 20 minutes
Servings: 5

Ingredients:

½ lb. Pork tenderloin
Nonstick cooking spray
2 Small heads of roasted garlic
Salt and ground black pepper

Directions:

Lightly spray all the sides of pork with cooking spray and then season with salt and black pepper. Now, rub the pork with roasted garlic.
Arrange the roast onto the lightly greased cooking tray.
Select "Air Fry" and the temperature to 400 °F. Set the time for 20 minutes and press "Start." When it shows "Turn Food," turn the pork.
Remove, then put the roast onto a platter for about 10 minutes before slicing. Slice and serve.

Nutrition:

Calories 238
Carbs 1.7g
Fat 1g
Protein 35.9g

142. Glazed Pork Tenderloin

Preparation time: 15 minutes
Cooking time: 20 minutes
Servings: 3

Ingredients:

1 lb. Pork tenderloin
2 tbsp Sriracha
2 tbsps. Honey
Salt, as required

Directions:

Insert the rotisserie rod through the pork tenderloin. Put the rotisserie forks, one on each side of the rod to secure the pork tenderloin.
In a small bowl, add the Sriracha, honey, and salt and mix well. Brush the pork tenderloin with the honey mixture evenly.
Select "Air Fry" to 350 °F.
Set the timer within 20 minutes and press "Start."
When done, press the red lever to release the rod.
Remove the pork and place it onto a platter for about 10 minutes before slicing. Cut the roast into desired-sized slices and serve.

Nutrition:

Calories 269
Carbs 13.5g
Fat 5.3g
Protein 39.7g

143. Buttered Pork Loin

Preparation time: 15 minutes
Cooking time: 30 minutes
Servings: 6

Ingredients:

2 lb. Pork loin
3 tbsp butter, melted and divided
Salt and ground black pepper

Directions:

Arrange a wire rack in a baking dish that will fit in the Air Fryer Oven. Coat the pork loin with melted butter evenly and then rub with salt and black pepper generously.
Arrange the pork loin into the prepared baking dish.
Choose "Air Fry" to 350 °F. Set the time for 30 minutes and press "Start." When it shows "Turn Food," do not turn the food.
Place the pork loin onto a cutting board. With a piece of foil, cover the pork loin for about 10 minutes before slicing. Slice the pork loin into desired-sized slices and serve.

Nutrition:

Calories 417
Carbs 0g
Fat 26.8g
Protein 41.4g

144. Spicy Pork Shoulder

Preparation time: 15 minutes
Cooking time: 55 minutes
Servings: 6

Ingredients:

1 tsp. ground cumin

1 tsp. Cayenne pepper
1 tsp. Garlic powder
Salt and ground black pepper
2 lbs. Skin-on pork shoulder

Directions:

In a small bowl, place spices, salt, and black pepper and mix well. Arrange the pork shoulder onto a cutting board, skin-side down.
Season the inner side of the pork shoulder with salt and black pepper. With kitchen twines, tie the pork shoulder into a long round cylinder shape.
Season the outer side of the pork shoulder with the spice mixture. Insert the rotisserie rod through the pork shoulder. Insert the rotisserie forks, one on each side of the rod to secure the pork shoulder.
Select "Roast" and then adjust the temperature to 350 °F.
Set the time for 55 minutes and press "Start." When it shows "Add Food," press the red lever down and load the rod's left side into the air fryer oven.
Now, slide the rod's left side into the groove along the metal bar, so it doesn't move. Then, close the door and touch "Rotate."
Remove the pork from the air fryer oven and place onto a platter for about 10 minutes before slicing.
With a sharp knife, cut the pork shoulder into desired-sized slices and serve.

Nutrition:

Calories 445
Carbs 0.7g
Fat 32.5g
Protein 35.4g

145. BBQ Pork Ribs

Preparation time: 15 minutes
Cooking time: 26 minutes
Servings: 4

Ingredients:

¼ cup Honey divided
¾ cup BBQ sauce
2 tbsps. Tomato ketchup
1 tbsp. Worcestershire sauce
1 tbsp. Soy sauce
½ tsp. Garlic powder
Ground white pepper
1¾ lbs. Pork ribs

Directions:

In a bowl, mix 3 tbsp of honey and the remaining ingredients except for the pork ribs. Add the pork ribs and coat with the mixture generously.
Refrigerate to marinate for about 20 minutes.
Arrange the ribs onto the greased cooking tray.
Select "Air Fry" to 355 °F. Set the time for 26 minutes and press "Start."
When the display shows "Turn Food," turn the ribs.
Transfer the ribs onto serving plates. Put the remaining honey and serve immediately.

Nutrition:

Calories 691
Carbs 37g
Fat 35.3g
Protein 53.1g

146. Cheeseburger Egg Rolls

Preparation time: 10 minutes
Cooking time: 7 minutes
Servings: 6

Ingredients:

6 egg roll wrappers
6 chopped dill pickle chips
1 tbsp. yellow mustard
3 tbsp. cream cheese
3 tbsp. shredded cheddar cheese
½ C. chopped onion
½ C. chopped bell pepper
¼ tsp onion powder
¼ tsp. garlic powder
8 ounces of raw lean ground beef

Directions:

Put the seasonings, beef, onion, and bell pepper in a skillet. Mix and crumble the beef until fully cooked.
Remove, then put the cream cheese, mustard, and cheddar cheese, mixing until melted.
Put the beef mixture into a large bowl and put the pickles.
Arrange the egg wrappers, then place 1/6th of beef batter into each one. Wet the egg roll wrapper edges slightly using water. Tuck sides to the middle and seals it with water.
Repeat the process with all the remaining egg rolls.
Place rolls into the air fryer, one batch at a time.
Set temperature to 392°F, and set time to 7 minutes.
Serve.

Nutrition:

Calories: 148
Carbs: 0g
Fat: 0g
Protein: 0g

147. Air Fried Grilled Steak

Preparation time: 5 minutes
Cooking time: 45 minutes
Servings: 2

Ingredients:

2 top sirloin steaks
3 tablespoons butter, melted
3 tablespoons olive oil
Salt and pepper to taste

Directions:

Preheat the air fryer oven for 5 minutes. Season the sirloin steaks with olive oil, salt, and pepper.
Put the beef in the air fryer basket—Cook for 45 minutes at 350°F.
Once cooked, serve with butter.

Nutrition:

Calories: 302
Carbs: 16g
Fat: 15g
Protein: 26g

148. Juicy Cheeseburgers

Preparation time: 5 minutes
Cooking time: 15 minutes
Servings: 4

Ingredients:

1 pound 93% lean ground beef
1 teaspoon Worcestershire sauce
1 tablespoon burger seasoning

Salt
Pepper
Cooking oil
4 slices cheese
buns

Directions:

Mix the ground beef, Worcestershire, burger seasoning, salt, and pepper to taste until well blended in a large bowl.

Grease the air fryer basket using cooking oil. You will need only a quick spritz. The burgers will produce oil as they cook. Shape the mixture into 4 patties.

Place the burgers in the air fryer. Set temperature to 375°F, and set time to 8 minutes.

Cook for 8 minutes. Flip the burgers. Cook again within 3 to 4 minutes.

Put a slice of cheese in each burger. Cook again in a minute, or until the cheese has melted. Serve on buns with any additional toppings of your choice.

Nutrition:

Calories: 249
Carbs: 24g
Fat: 11g
Protein: 12g

149. Beef Brisket Recipe from Texas

Preparation time: 15 minutes
Cooking time: 1 hour & 30 minutes
Servings: 8

Ingredients:

1 ½ cup beef stock
1 bay leaf
1 tablespoon garlic powder
1 tablespoon onion powder
2 pounds beef brisket, trimmed
2 tablespoons chili powder
2 teaspoons dry mustard
4 tablespoons olive oil
Salt and pepper to taste

Directions:

Preheat the air fryer oven for 5 minutes. Put all the fixings in a deep baking dish that will fit in the air fryer.

Bake for 1 hour and 30 minutes at 400°F. Stir the beef every after 30 minutes to soak in the sauce.

Nutrition:

Calories: 170
Carbs: 0g
Fat: 6g
Protein: 28g

150. Copycat Taco Bell Crunch Wraps

Preparation time: 15 minutes
Cooking time: 2 minutes
Servings: 6

Ingredients:

6 wheat tostadas
2 C. sour cream
2 C. Mexican blend cheese
2 C. shredded lettuce
12 ounces low-sodium nacho cheese
3 Roma tomatoes
6 12-inch wheat tortillas
1 1/3 C. water
2 packets low-sodium taco seasoning
2 pounds of lean ground beef

Directions:

Ensure your air fryer is preheated to 400 degrees.

Make beef according to taco seasoning packets.

Place 2/3 cup prepared beef, 4 tbsp cheese, 1 tostada, 1/3 cup sour cream, 1/3 cup lettuce, 1/6 of tomatoes, and 1/3 cup cheese on each tortilla.

Fold up tortillas edges and repeat with remaining ingredients. Lay the folded sides of tortillas down into the air fryer and spray with olive oil.

Set temperature to 400°F, and set time to 2 minutes.

Cook 2 minutes till browned.

Nutrition:

Calories: 530
Carbs: 71g
Fat: 21g
Protein: 16g

151. Steak and Mushroom Gravy

Preparation time: 15 minutes
Cooking time: 15 minutes
Servings: 4

Ingredients:

4 cubed steaks
2 large eggs
1/2 dozen mushrooms
4 tablespoons unsalted butter
4 tablespoons black pepper
2 tablespoons salt
1/2 teaspoon onion powder
1/2 teaspoon garlic powder
1/4 teaspoon cayenne powder
1 1/4 teaspoons paprika
1 1/2 cups whole milk
1/3 cup flour
tablespoons vegetable oil

Directions:

Mix half of the flour and a pinch of black pepper in a shallow bowl or on a plate.

Beat 2 eggs in a bowl and mix in a pinch of salt and pepper.

Mix the other half of the flour with pepper to taste, garlic powder, paprika, cayenne, and onion powder in a separate shallow bowl.

Chop mushrooms and set aside.

Press your steak into the first flour mixture, then dip in egg, then press the steak into the second flour mixture until covered completely.

Set temperature to 360°F, and set time to 15 minutes, flipping halfway through.

While the steak cooks, warm the butter over medium heat and add mushrooms to sauté.

Add 4 tablespoons of the flour and pepper mix to the pan and mix until there are no clumps of flour.

Mix in whole milk and simmer. Serve over steak for breakfast, lunch, or dinner.

Nutrition:

Calories: 188
Carbs: 9g
Fat: 5g
Protein: 29g

152. Chimichurri Skirt Steak

Preparation time: 10 minutes
Cooking time: 8 minutes
Servings: 2

Ingredients:

2 x 8 oz Skirt Steak
1 cup Finely Chopped Parsley
¼ cup Finely Chopped Mint
2 Tbsp Fresh Oregano (Washed & finely chopped)
3 Finely Chopped Cloves of Garlic
1 Tsp Red Pepper Flakes (Crushed)
1 Tbsp Ground Cumin
1 Tsp Cayenne Pepper
2 Tsp Smoked Paprika
1 Tsp Salt
¼ Tsp Pepper
¾ cup Oil
3 Tbsp Red Wine Vinegar

Directions:

Throw all the ingredients in a bowl (besides the steak) and mix well.
Put ¼ cup of the mixture in a plastic baggie with the steak and leave in the fridge overnight.
Leave the bag out at room temperature for at least 30 min before popping into the air fryer. Preheat for a minute or two to 390° F before cooking until med-rare (8–10 min).
Set temperature to 390°F, and set time to 10 minutes.
Put 2 Tbsp of the chimichurri mix on top of each steak before serving.

Nutrition:

Calories: 250
Carbs: 3g
Fat: 19g
Protein: 17g

153. Country Fried Steak

Preparation time: 5 minutes
Cooking time: 12 minutes
Servings: 2

Ingredients:

1 tsp. pepper
2 C. almond milk
2 tbsp. almond flour
6 ounces ground sausage meat
1 tsp. pepper
1 tsp. salt
1 tsp. garlic powder
1 tsp. onion powder
1 C. panko breadcrumbs
1 C. almond flour
3 beaten eggs
6 ounces sirloin steak, pounded till thin

Directions:

Season panko breadcrumbs with spices. Dredge steak in flour, then egg, and then seasoned panko mixture.
Place into an air fryer basket. Set temperature to 370°F, and set time to 12 minutes.
To make sausage gravy, cook sausage and drain off fat, but reserve 2 tablespoons.
Add flour to sausage and mix until incorporated.
Gradually mix in milk over medium to high heat until it becomes thick.
Season mixture with pepper and cook 3 minutes longer. Serve steak topped with gravy and enjoy.

Nutrition:

Calories: 250
Carbs: 13g
Fat: 17g
Protein: 9g

154. Creamy Burger & Potato Bake

Preparation time: 5 minutes
Cooking time: 55 minutes
Servings: 3

Ingredients:

salt to taste
freshly ground pepper, to taste
1/2 (10.75 ounces) can condense cream of mushroom soup
1/2-pound lean ground beef
1-1/2 cups peeled and thinly sliced potatoes
1/2 cup shredded Cheddar cheese
1/4 cup chopped onion
1/4 cup and 2 tablespoons milk

Directions:

Lightly grease baking pan of the air fryer with cooking spray. Add ground beef. For 10 minutes, cook at 360°F. Stir and crumble halfway through cooking time.
Meanwhile, in a bowl, whisk well pepper, salt, milk, onion, and mushroom soup. Mix well.
Drain fat off ground beef and transfer beef to a plate.
In the same air fryer baking pan, layer ½ of potatoes on the bottom, then ½ of soup mixture, and then ½ of beef. Repeat process.
Cover pan with foil. Cook for 30 minutes. Remove the foil and cook again within 15 minutes or until potatoes are tender. Serve and enjoy.

Nutrition:

Calories: 103
Carbs: 4g
Fat: 9g
Protein: 2g

155. Beefy 'n Cheesy Spanish Rice Casserole

Preparation time: 15 minutes
Cooking time: 50 minutes
Servings: 3

Ingredients:

2 tablespoons chopped green bell pepper
1 tablespoon chopped fresh cilantro
1/2-pound lean ground beef
1/2 cup water
1/2 teaspoon salt
1/2 teaspoon brown sugar
1/2 pinch ground black pepper
1/3 cup uncooked long-grain rice
1/4 cup finely chopped onion
1/4 cup Chile sauce
1/4 teaspoon ground cumin
1/4 teaspoon Worcestershire sauce
1/4 cup shredded Cheddar cheese
1/2 (14.5 ounces) can canned tomatoes

Directions:

Lightly grease baking pan of the air fryer with cooking spray. Add ground beef.

For 10 minutes, cook at 360°F. Halfway through cooking time, stir and crumble beef. Discard excess fat.
Stir in pepper, Worcestershire sauce, cumin, brown sugar, salt, Chile sauce, rice, water, tomatoes, green bell pepper, and onion.
Mix well. Cover the pan using a foil and cook for 25 minutes, stirring occasionally.
Give it one last good stir, press down firmly, and sprinkle cheese on top. Cook uncovered for 15 minutes at 390°F until tops are lightly browned.
Serve and enjoy with chopped cilantro.
Nutrition:
Calories: 371
Carbs: 30g
Fat: 13g
Protein: 30g

156. Warming Winter Beef with Celery

Preparation time: 5 minutes
Cooking time: 12 minutes
Servings: 4
Ingredients:
9 ounces tender beef, chopped
1/2 cup leeks, chopped
1/2 cup celery stalks, chopped
2 cloves garlic, smashed
2 tablespoons red cooking wine
3/4 cup cream of celery soup
2 sprigs rosemary, chopped
1/4 teaspoon smoked paprika
3/4 teaspoons salt
1/4 teaspoon black pepper
Directions:
Add the beef, leeks, celery, and garlic to the baking dish; cook for about 5 minutes at 390 degrees F.
Once the meat is starting to tender, pour in the wine and soup—season with rosemary, smoked paprika, salt, and black pepper. Now, cook an additional 7 minutes.
Nutrition:
Calories: 125
Carbs: 0g
Fat: 0g
Protein: 0g

157. Beef & Veggie Spring Rolls

Preparation time: 15 minutes
Cooking time: 12 minutes
Servings: 10
Ingredients:
2-ounce Asian rice noodles
1 tablespoon sesame oil
7-ounce ground beef
1 small onion, chopped
3 garlic cloves, crushed
1 cup of fresh mixed vegetables
1 teaspoon soy sauce
1 packet spring roll skins
2 tablespoons water
Olive oil, as required
Directions:
Dip the noodles in warm water until soft.
Drain and cut into small lengths. Heat the oil in a pan and add the onion and garlic and sauté for about 4-5 minutes.
Add beef and cook for about 4-5 minutes. Add vegetables and cook for about 5-7 minutes or till cooked through.
Stir in soy sauce and remove from the heat. Stir in the noodles and keep aside till all the juices have been absorbed.
Preheat the air fryer oven to 350 degrees F. Place the spring rolls skin onto a smooth surface.
Add a line of the filling diagonally across. Fold the top point over the filling and then fold in both sides.
On the final point, brush it with water before rolling to seal. Brush the spring rolls with oil.
Arrange the rolls in batches in the air fryer and Cook for about 8 minutes. Repeat with remaining rolls.
Now, place spring rolls onto a baking sheet—Bake for about 6 minutes per side.
Nutrition:
Calories: 160
Carbs: 0g
Fat: 0g
Protein: 0g

158. Charred Onions and Steak Cube BBQ

Preparation time: 5 minutes
Cooking time: 40 minutes
Servings: 3
Ingredients:
1 cup red onions, cut into wedges
1 tablespoon dry mustard
1 tablespoon olive oil
1-pound boneless beef sirloin, cut into cubes
Salt and pepper to taste
Directions:
Preheat the air fryer to 390°F. Place the grill pan accessory in the air fryer.
Toss all the fixings in a bowl and mix until everything is coated with the seasonings.
Put on the grill pan and cook for 40 minutes. Halfway through the cooking time, give a stir to cook evenly.
Nutrition:
Calories: 120
Carbs: 0g
Fat: 0g
Protein: 18g

159. Beef Stroganoff

Preparation time: 15 minutes
Cooking time: 14 minutes
Servings: 4
Ingredients:
9 oz. Tender Beef
1 Onion, chopped
1 Tbsp Paprika
3/4 Cup Sour Cream
Salt and pepper to taste
Baking Dish
Directions:
Preheat the air fryer oven to 390 degrees. Slice the beef, then marinate it with the paprika.
Add the chopped onions into the baking dish and heat for about 2 minutes in the air fryer oven.

When the onions are transparent, add the beef into the dish and cook for 5 minutes.
Once the beef is starting to tender, pour in the sour cream and cook for another 7 minutes.
Season with salt and pepper and serve.

Nutrition:
Calories: 127
Carbs: 9g
Fat: 9g
Protein: 6g

160. Cheesy Ground Beef and Mac Taco Casserole

Preparation time: 15 minutes
Cooking time: 25 minutes
Servings: 5

Ingredients:
1-ounce shredded Cheddar cheese
1-ounce shredded Monterey Jack cheese
2 tablespoons chopped green onions
1/2 (10.75 ounces) can condensed tomato soup
1/2-pound lean ground beef
1/2 cup crushed tortilla chips
1/4-pound macaroni, cooked according to manufacturer's Instructions
1/4 cup chopped onion
1/4 cup sour cream (optional)
1/2 (1.25 ounce) package taco seasoning mix
1/2 can diced tomatoes

Directions:
Lightly grease baking pan of the air fryer with cooking spray. Add onion and ground beef. For 10 minutes, cook at 360°F. Halfway through cooking time, stir and crumble ground beef.
Add taco seasoning, diced tomatoes, and tomato soup. Mix well. Mix in pasta.
Sprinkle crushed tortilla chips. Sprinkle cheese.
Cook for 15 minutes at 390°F until tops are lightly browned, and cheese is melted.
Serve and enjoy.

Nutrition:
Calories: 225
Carbs: 16g
Fat: 8g
Protein: 25g

161. Ham and Cheese Rollups

Preparation time: 5 minutes
Cooking time: 8 minutes
Servings: 12

Ingredients:
2 tsp. raw honey
2 tsp. dried parsley
1 tbsp. poppy seeds
½ C. melted coconut oil
¼ C. spicy brown mustard
9 slices of provolone cheese
10 ounces of thinly sliced Black Forest Ham
1 tube of crescent rolls

Directions:
Roll out dough into a rectangle. Spread 2-3 tablespoons of spicy mustard onto the dough, then layer provolone cheese and ham slices. Roll the filled dough up as tight as you can and slice into 12-15 pieces.
Melt coconut oil and mix with a pinch of salt and pepper, parsley, honey, and the rest of the mustard. Brush mustard mixture over roll-ups and sprinkle with poppy seeds. Grease the air fryer oven basket liberally with olive oil and add roll-ups.
Set oven to Air Fry at 350°F, and set time to 8 minutes. Serve.

Nutrition:
Calories: 280
Carbs: 27g
Fat: 13g
Protein: 13g

162. Pork Taquitos

Preparation time: 15 minutes
Cooking time: 16 minutes
Servings: 8

Ingredients:
1 juiced lime
10 whole-wheat tortillas
2 ½ C. shredded mozzarella cheese
30 ounces of cooked and shredded pork tenderloin

Directions:
Ensure your air fryer oven is preheated to 380 degrees. Drizzle pork with lime juice and gently mix. Warm the tortillas in the microwave with a dampened paper towel to soften. Add about 3 ounces of pork and ¼ cup of shredded cheese to each tortilla. Tightly roll them up. Spray the air fryer oven basket with a bit of olive oil.
Set oven to Air Fry at 380°F, and set time to 10 minutes. Air fry taquitos 7-10 minutes till tortillas turn a slight golden color, making sure to flip halfway through the cooking process.

Nutrition:
Calories: 210
Carbs: 25g
Fat: 9g
Protein: 7g

163. Juicy Pork Ribs Ole

Preparation time: 15 minutes
Cooking time: 25 minutes
Servings: 4

Ingredients:
1 rack of pork ribs
1/2 cup low-fat milk
1 tablespoon taco seasoning mix
1 can tomato sauce
1/2 teaspoon ground black pepper
1 teaspoon seasoned salt
1 tablespoon cornstarch
1 teaspoon canola oil

Directions:
Place all ingredients in a mixing dish; let them marinate for 1 hour.
Cook the marinated ribs approximately 25 minutes at 390 degrees F. Work with batches.
Enjoy

Nutrition:
Calories: 240
Carbs: 0g

Fat: 17g
Protein: 54g

164. Pork Tenders with Bell Peppers

Preparation time: 15 minutes
Cooking time: 15 minutes
Servings: 4
Ingredients:
11 oz Pork Tenderloin
1 Bell Pepper, in thin strips
1 Red Onion, sliced
2 tsp. Provencal Herbs
Black Pepper to taste
1 tbsp Olive Oil
1/2 tbsp Mustard
Directions:
Preheat the Air fryer oven to 390 degrees.
In the oven dish, mix the bell pepper strips with the onion, herbs, and salt plus pepper to taste.
Put half a tablespoon of olive oil to the batter.
Slice the pork tenderloin into four pieces and rub with salt, pepper, and mustard.
Thinly coat the pieces with remaining olive oil and place them upright in the oven pan on top of the pepper mixture.
Set it to 15 minutes, then roast the meat and the vegetables. Turn the pork meat and mix the peppers halfway through. Serve with a fresh salad.
Nutrition:
Calories: 310
Carbs: 30g
Fat: 9g
Protein: 28g

165. Cajun Bacon Pork Loin Fillet

Preparation time: 1 hour & 15 minutes
Cooking time: 20 minutes
Servings: 6
Ingredients:
1½ pounds pork loin fillet or pork tenderloin
3 tablespoons olive oil
2 tablespoons Cajun Spice Mix
Salt
6 slices bacon
Olive oil spray
Directions:
Slice the pork in half so that it will fit in the air fryer basket.
Place both pieces of meat in a resealable plastic bag. Add the oil, Cajun seasoning, and salt to taste, if using. Seal the bag and massage to coat all of the meat with the oil and seasonings. Marinate in the fridge within 1 hour or up to 24 hours.
Remove the pork from the bag and wrap 3 bacon slices around each piece. Spray the Air Fryer Oven basket with olive oil spray. Place the meat in the Air Fryer Oven basket.
Set oven to Air Fry at 350°F for 15 minutes. Increase the temperature to 400°F for 5 minutes. Use a meat thermometer to ensure the meat has reached an internal temperature of 145°F.
Let the meat rest for 10 minutes. Slice into 6 medallions and serve.
Nutrition:
Calories: 190
Carbs: 5g
Fat: 9g
Protein: 23g

166. Scotch Eggs

Preparation time: 15 minutes
Cooking time: 15 minutes
Servings: 8
Ingredients:
2 pounds ground pork or ground beef
2 teaspoons sea salt
½ teaspoon ground black pepper
8 large hard-boiled eggs, peeled
2 cups of pork dust
Dijon mustard, for serving (optional)
Directions:
Spray the Air Fryer Oven basket using the avocado oil.
Preheat the air fryer oven to 400°F.
Put the ground pork in a bowl, put the salt and pepper, and use your hands to mix until seasoned throughout.
Flatten about ¼ pound of ground pork in the palm of your hand and place a peeled egg in the center. Fold the pork entirely around the egg.
Repeat with the remaining eggs. Place the pork dust in a medium-sized bowl.
One at a time, roll the ground pork–covered eggs in the pork dust and use your hands to press it into the eggs to form a nice crust.
Place the eggs in the Air Fryer Oven basket and spray them with avocado oil.
Set oven to Air Fry at 400°F. Cook the eggs for 15 minutes, or until the pork's internal temperature reaches 145°F and the outside is golden brown.
Garnish with ground black pepper and serve with Dijon mustard, if desired.
Nutrition:
Calories: 306
Carbs: 20g
Fat: 19g
Protein: 12g

167. Asian Pork Chops

Preparation time: 2 hours & 15 minutes
Cooking time: 15 minutes
Servings: 4
Ingredients:
1/2 cup hoisin sauce
3 tablespoons cider vinegar
1 tablespoon Asian sweet chili sauce
1/4 teaspoon garlic powder
4 (1/2-inch-thick) boneless pork chops
1 teaspoon salt
1/2 teaspoon pepper
Directions:
Stir hoisin, chili sauce, garlic powder, plus vinegar in a mixing bowl.
Separate 1/4 cup of this batter, add pork chops to the bowl and marinate in the fridge for 2 hours. Remove the pork chops and place them on a plate.
Sprinkle each side of the pork chop evenly with salt and pepper.

Cook at 360 degrees for 14 minutes, flipping halfway through.

Nutrition:

Calories: 359
Carbs: 5g
Fat: 8g
Protein: 50g

168. BBQ Riblets

Preparation time: 15 minutes
Cooking time: 25 minutes
Servings: 4

Ingredients:

1 rack pork riblets, cut into individual riblets
1 teaspoon fine sea salt
1 teaspoon ground black pepper
Sauce:
¼ cup apple cider vinegar
¼ cup beef broth
¼ cup Swerve confectioners'-style sweetener or powdered sweetener
¼ cup tomato sauce
1 teaspoon liquid smoke
1 teaspoon onion powder
2 cloves garlic, minced

Directions:

Spray the Air Fryer Oven basket with avocado oil. Preheat the air fryer oven to 350°F. Season the riblets well on all sides with the salt and pepper. Place the riblets in the air fryer basket, then onto the Baking Pan. Set oven to Air Fry at 350°F, and cook for 10 minutes, flipping halfway through.
While the riblets cook, mix all the sauce ingredients in a 6-inch pie pan.
Remove the riblets, and place them in the pie pan with the sauce. Stir to coat the riblets in the sauce. Transfer the pan to the Air Fryer Oven and cook for 10 to 15 minutes, until the pork is cooked through and the internal temperature reaches 145°F. Serve.

Nutrition:

Calories: 220
Carbs: 35g
Fat: 4g
Protein: 18g

169. Bacon-Wrapped Stuffed Pork Chops

Preparation time: 15 minutes
Cooking time: 20 minutes
Servings: 4

Ingredients:

4 (1-inch-thick) boneless pork chops
2 (5.2-ounce) packages Boursin cheese
8 slices thin-cut bacon

Directions:

Grease the Air Fryer Oven basket with avocado oil. Preheat the air fryer oven to 400°F.
Place one of the chops on a cutting board. Make a 1-inch-wide incision on the top edge of the chop. Carefully cut into the chop to form a large pocket, leaving a ½-inch border along the sides and bottom. Repeat with the other 3 chops. Snip the corner of a large resealable plastic bag to form a ¾-inch hole.
Place the Boursin cheese in the bag and pipe the cheese into the pockets in the chops, dividing the cheese evenly among them.
Wrap 2 slices of bacon around each chop and secure the ends with toothpicks.
Place the bacon-wrapped chops in the Air Fryer Oven basket. Set oven to Air Fry at 400°F and cook for 10 minutes, then flip the chops and cook for another 8 to 10 minutes, until the bacon is crisp, the chops are cooked through, and the internal temperature reaches 145°F.

Nutrition:

Calories: 150
Carbs: 1g
Fat: 6g
Protein: 22g

170. Panko-Breaded Pork Chops

Preparation time: 15 minutes
Cooking time: 12 minutes
Servings: 6

Ingredients:

5 (3½- to 5-ounce) pork chops
Seasoning salt
Pepper
¼ cup all-purpose flour
2 tablespoons panko bread crumbs
Cooking oil

Directions:

Rub the pork chops using a salt and pepper to taste.
Put the flour on both sides of the pork chops, then coat both sides with panko bread crumbs.
Put the pork chops in the air fryer basket. Stacking them is okay.
Spray the pork chops with cooking oil. Set oven to Air Fry at 400°F. Cook for 6 minutes.
Flip the pork chops. Cook for an additional 6 minutes. Cool before serving.

Nutrition:

Calories: 253
Carbs: 7g
Fat: 14g
Protein: 26g

171. Cajun Pork Steaks

Preparation time: 15 minutes
Cooking time: 20 minutes
Servings: 6

Ingredients:

4-6 pork steaks
BBQ sauce:
Cajun seasoning
1 tbsp. vinegar
1 tsp. low-sodium soy sauce
½ C. brown sugar
½ C. vegan ketchup

Directions:

Ensure your air fryer oven is preheated to 290 degrees. Sprinkle pork steaks with Cajun seasoning. Combine remaining ingredients and brush onto steaks. Add coated steaks to Air Fryer Oven basket. Set oven to "Air Fry" at 290°F, and set time to 20 minutes. Cook 15-20 minutes till just browned.

Nutrition:

Calories: 229
Carbs: 2g
Fat: 10g
Protein: 32g

172. Porchetta-Style Pork Chops

Preparation time: 15 minutes
Cooking time: 15 minutes
Servings: 2

Ingredients:

1 tablespoon extra-virgin olive oil
Grated zest of 1 lemon
2 cloves garlic, minced
2 teaspoons chopped fresh rosemary
1 teaspoon finely chopped fresh sage
1 teaspoon fennel seeds, lightly crushed
¼ to ½ teaspoon red pepper flakes
1 teaspoon kosher salt
1 teaspoon black pepper
(8-ounce) center-cut bone-in pork chops, about 1 inch thick

Directions:

In a small bowl, combine the olive oil, zest, garlic, rosemary, sage, fennel seeds, red pepper, salt, and black pepper.
Stir, crushing the herbs with the back of a spoon, until a paste form. Rub the seasoning mix on each side of the pork chops.
Put the chops inside the air fryer basket—set oven to "Air Fry" at 375°F for 15 minutes. Serve.

Nutrition:

Calories: 250
Carbs: 15g
Fat: 9g
Protein: 34g

173. Dry Rub Baby Back Ribs

Preparation time: 15 minutes
Cooking time: 35 minutes
Servings: 2

Ingredients:

2 teaspoons fine sea salt
1 teaspoon ground black pepper
2 teaspoons smoked paprika
1 teaspoon garlic powder
1 teaspoon onion powder
½ teaspoon chili powder (optional)
1 rack baby back ribs, half crosswise

Directions:

Grease your Air Fryer Oven basket with avocado oil. Preheat the air fryer oven to 350°F. Mix the salt, pepper, and seasonings in a small bowl. Season the ribs on all sides with the seasoning mixture.
Place the ribs in the air fryer basket, then set oven to Air Fry at 350°F, cook for 15 minutes, then flip the ribs over and cook for another 15 to 20 minutes.

Nutrition:

Calories: 64
Carbs: 15g
Fat: 1g
Protein: 1g

174. Pork Milanese

Preparation time: 15 minutes
Cooking time: 12 minutes
Servings: 4

Ingredients:

4 (1-inch) boneless pork chops
Fine sea salt and ground black pepper
2 large eggs
¾ cup powdered Parmesan cheese about 2¼ ounces
Chopped fresh parsley, for garnish
Lemon slices, for serving

Directions:

Spray the air fryer basket using avocado oil. Preheat the air fryer oven to 400°F.
Put the pork chops in the middle of 2 sheets of plastic wrap and pound them with the flat side of a meat tenderizer until they're ¼ inch thick.
Lightly season both sides of the chops with salt and pepper. Lightly beat the eggs in a shallow bowl.
Divide the Parmesan cheese evenly between 2 bowls and set the bowls in this order: Parmesan, eggs, Parmesan.
Dredge a chop in the first bowl of Parmesan, then dip it in the eggs, and then dredge it again in the second bowl of Parmesan, making sure both sides and all edges are well coated. Repeat with the remaining chops.
Place the chops in the Air Fryer Oven basket and cook for 12 minutes, or until the internal temperature reaches 145°F, flipping halfway through.
Garnish with fresh parsley, then serve with lemon slices.

Nutrition:

Calories: 200
Carbs: 15g
Fat: 5g
Protein: 21g

175. Roasted Pork Tenderloin

Preparation time: 15 minutes
Cooking time: 1 hour
Servings: 4

Ingredients:

1 (3-pound) pork tenderloin
2 tablespoons extra-virgin olive oil
2 garlic cloves, minced
1 teaspoon dried basil
1 teaspoon dried oregano
1 teaspoon dried thyme
Salt
Pepper

Directions:

Greased the pork tenderloin with the olive oil.
Massage the garlic, basil, oregano, thyme, and salt and pepper to taste all over the tenderloin.
Place the tenderloin in the Air fryer basket. Set oven to "Air Fry" at 400°F. Cook for 45 minutes. Use a meat thermometer to test for doneness.
Open the oven and flip the pork tenderloin—Cook for an additional 15 minutes. Remove the cooked pork from the Air Fryer Oven and allow it to rest for 10 minutes before cutting.

Nutrition:

Calories: 46
Carbs: 0g
Fat: 1g

Protein: 8g

176. Juicy Pork Chops

Preparation Time: 10 minutes
Cooking Time: 16 minutes
Servings: 4
Ingredients:
4 pork chops, boneless
2 tsp olive oil
½ tsp celery seed
½ tsp parsley
½ tsp granulated onion
½ tsp granulated garlic
¼ tsp sugar
½ tsp salt
Directions:
In a small bowl, mix oil, celery seed, parsley, granulated onion, granulated garlic, sugar, and salt.
Rub seasoning mixture all over the pork chops.
Place pork chops on the air fryer oven pan and cook at 350 F for 8 minutes.
Turn pork chops on its other side and cook for 8 minutes more.
Serve and enjoy.
Nutrition:
Calories 279
Fat 22.3 g
Carbohydrates 0.6 g
Sugar 0.3 g
Protein 18.1 g
Cholesterol 69 mg

177. Crispy Meatballs

Preparation Time: 10 minutes
Cooking Time: 12 minutes
Servings: 8
Ingredients:
1 lb. ground pork
1 lb. ground beef
1 tbsp Worcestershire sauce
½ cup feta cheese, crumbled
½ cup breadcrumbs
2 eggs, lightly beaten
¼ cup fresh parsley, chopped
1 tbsp garlic, minced
1 onion, chopped
¼ tsp pepper
1 tsp salt
Directions:
Put all the fixings into the mixing bowl and mix until well combined.
Spray the tray pan with cooking spray.
Make small balls from meat mixture and arrange on a pan and air fry t 400 F for 10-12 minutes.
Serve and enjoy.
Nutrition:
Calories 263
Fat 9 g
Carbohydrates 7.5 g
Sugar 1.9 g
Protein 35.9 g
Cholesterol 141 mg

178. Flavorful Steak

Preparation Time: 10 minutes
Cooking Time: 18 minutes
Servings: 2
Ingredients:
2 steaks, rinsed and pat dry
½ tsp garlic powder
1 tsp olive oil
Pepper
Salt
Directions:
Massage the steaks with olive oil and season with garlic powder, pepper, and salt.
Preheat the air fryer oven to 400 F.
Place steaks on air fryer oven pan and air fry for 10-18 minutes. Turn halfway through.
Serve and enjoy.
Nutrition:
Calories 361
Fat 10.9 g
Carbohydrates 0.5 g
Sugar 0.2 g
Protein 61.6 g
Cholesterol 153 mg

179. Lemon Garlic Lamb Chops

Preparation Time: 10 minutes
Cooking Time: 6 minutes
Servings: 6
Ingredients:
6 lamb loin chops
2 tbsp fresh lemon juice
1 ½ tbsp lemon zest
1 tbsp dried rosemary
1 tbsp olive oil
1 tbsp garlic, minced
Pepper
Salt
Directions:
Add lamb chops in a mixing bowl.
Add remaining ingredients on top of lamb chops and coat well.
Arrange the meat lambs on the air fryer oven tray and air fry at 400 F within 3 minutes.
Turn lamb chops to another side and air fry for 3 minutes more.
Serve and enjoy.
Nutrition:
Calories 69
Fat 6 g
Carbohydrates 1.2 g
Sugar 0.2 g
Protein 3 g
Cholesterol 0 mg

180. Honey Mustard Pork Tenderloin

Preparation Time: 10 minutes
Cooking Time: 26 minutes
Servings: 4
Ingredients:
1 lb. pork tenderloin
1 tsp sriracha sauce
1 tbsp garlic, minced
2 tbsp soy sauce
1 ½ tbsp honey

¾ tbsp Dijon mustard
1 tbsp mustard

Directions:

Add sriracha sauce, garlic, soy sauce, honey, Dijon mustard, and mustard into the large zip-lock bag and mix well.
Add pork tenderloin into the bag. Seal, then place it in the refrigerator overnight.
Preheat the air fryer oven to 380 F.
Spray the air fryer tray with cooking spray, then place marinated pork tenderloin on a tray and air fry for 26 minutes. Turn pork tenderloin after every 5 minutes.
Slice and serve.

Nutrition:

Calories 195
Fat 4.1 g
Carbohydrates 8 g
Sugar 6.7 g
Protein 30.5 g
Cholesterol 83 mg

181. Easy Rosemary Lamb Chops

Preparation Time: 10 minutes
Cooking Time: 6 minutes
Servings: 4

Ingredients:

4 lamb chops
2 tbsp dried rosemary
¼ cup fresh lemon juice
Pepper
Salt

Directions:

In a small bowl, mix lemon juice, rosemary, pepper, and salt.
Brush the lemon juice rosemary mixture over lamb chops.
Place lamb chops on air fryer oven tray and air fry setting at 400 F for 3 minutes.
Turn lamb chops to the other side and cook for 3 minutes more.
Serve and enjoy.

Nutrition:

Calories 267
Fat 21.7 g
Carbohydrates 1.4 g
Sugar 0.3 g
Protein 16.9 g
Cholesterol 0 mg

182. Juicy Steak Bites

Preparation Time: 10 minutes
Cooking Time: 9 minutes
Servings: 4

Ingredients:

1 lb. sirloin steak, cut into bite-size pieces
1 tbsp steak seasoning
1 tbsp olive oil
Pepper
Salt

Directions:

Preheat the air fryer oven to 390 F.
Add steak pieces into the large mixing bowl. Add steak seasoning, oil, pepper, and salt over steak pieces and toss until well coated.
Transfer steak pieces to air fryer pan and air fry for 5 minutes.
Turn the steak pieces to the other side and cook for 4 minutes more. Serve and enjoy.

Nutrition:

Calories 241
Fat 10.6 g
Carbohydrates 0 g
Sugar 0 g
Protein 34.4 g
Cholesterol 101 mg

183. Greek Lamb Chops

Preparation Time: 10 minutes
Cooking Time: 10 minutes
Servings: 4

Ingredients:

2 lbs. lamb chops
2 tsp garlic, minced
1 ½ tsp dried oregano
¼ cup fresh lemon juice
¼ cup olive oil
½ tsp pepper
1 tsp salt

Directions:

Add lamb chops in a mixing bowl. Add remaining ingredients over the lamb chops and coat well.
Arrange lamb chops on the air fryer oven tray and cook at 400 F for 5 minutes.
Turn lamb chops and cook for 5 minutes more.
Serve and enjoy.

Nutrition:

Calories 538
Fat 29.4 g
Carbohydrates 1.3 g
Sugar 0.4 g
Protein 64 g
Cholesterol 204 mg

184. Easy Beef Roast

Preparation Time: 10 minutes
Cooking Time: 45 minutes
Servings: 6

Ingredients:

2 ½ lbs. beef roast
2 tbsp Italian seasoning

Directions:

Arrange roast on the rotisserie spite.
Rub roast with Italian seasoning then insert into the air fryer oven.
Air fry at 350 F for 45 minutes or until the roast's internal temperature reaches 145 F.
Slice and serve.

Nutrition:

Calories 365
Fat 13.2 g
Carbohydrates 0.5 g
Sugar 0.4 g
Protein 57.4 g
Cholesterol 172 mg

185. Herb Butter Rib-eye Steak

Preparation Time: 10 minutes
Cooking Time: 14 minutes
Servings: 4

Ingredients:

2 lb. rib eye steak, bone-in
1 tsp fresh rosemary, chopped
1 tsp fresh thyme, chopped
1 tsp fresh chives, chopped
2 tsp fresh parsley, chopped
1 tsp garlic, minced
¼ cup butter softened
Pepper
Salt

Directions:

Mix the butter plus herbs in a small bowl.
Rub herb butter on rib-eye steak and place it in the refrigerator for 30 minutes.
Place marinated steak on air fryer oven pan and cook at 400 F for 12-14 minutes.
Serve and enjoy.

Nutrition:

Calories 416
Fat 36.7 g
Carbohydrates 0.7 g
Sugar 0 g
Protein 20.3 g
Cholesterol 106 mg

186. BBQ Pork Chops

Preparation Time: 10 minutes
Cooking Time: 7 minutes
Servings: 4

Ingredients:

4 pork chops
For rub:
½ tsp allspice
½ tsp dry mustard
1 tsp ground cumin
1 tsp garlic powder
½ tsp chili powder
½ tsp paprika
1 tbsp brown sugar
1 tsp salt

Directions:

Mix all the rub fixings in a small bowl and rub all over pork chops.
Arrange pork chops on air fryer tray and air fry at 400 F for 5.
Turn pork chops on its other side and air fry for 2 minutes more.
Serve and enjoy.

Nutrition:

Calories 273
Fat 20.2 g
Carbohydrates 3.4 g
Sugar 2.4 g
Protein 18.4 g
Cholesterol 69 mg

187. Simple Beef Patties

Preparation Time: 10 minutes
Cooking Time: 13 minutes
Servings: 4

Ingredients:

1 lb. ground beef
½ tsp garlic powder
¼ tsp onion powder
Pepper
Salt

Directions:

Preheat the air fryer oven to 400 F.
Add ground meat, garlic powder, onion powder, pepper, and salt into the mixing bowl and mix until well combined.
Make even shape patties from meat mixture and arrange at air fryer pan.
Cook patties for 10 minutes. Turn patties after 5 minutes. Serve and enjoy.

Nutrition:

Calories 212
Fat 7.1 g
Carbohydrates 0.4 g
Sugar 0.1 g
Protein 34.5 g
Cholesterol 101 mg

188. Marinated Pork Chops

Preparation Time: 10 minutes
Cooking Time: 30 minutes
Servings: 2

Ingredients:

2 pork chops, boneless
1 tsp garlic powder
½ cup flour
1 cup buttermilk
Pepper
Salt

Directions:

Add pork chops and buttermilk in a zip-lock bag. Seal the bag and place it properly in the refrigerator overnight.
In another zip-lock bag, add flour, garlic powder, pepper, and salt.
Remove marinated pork chops from buttermilk and add in flour mixture and shake until well coated.
Preheat the air fryer oven to 380 F.
Grease air fryer tray with cooking spray.
Arrange pork chops on a tray and air fryer for 28-30 minutes.
Turn pork chops after 18 minutes. Serve and enjoy.

Nutrition:

Calories 424
Fat 21.3 g
Carbohydrates 30.8 g
Sugar 6.3 g
Protein 25.5 g
Cholesterol 74 mg

189. Pork Satay

Preparation time: 15 minutes
Cooking time: 14 minutes
Servings: 4

Ingredients:

1 (1-pound) pork tenderloin, cut into 1½-inch cubes
¼ cup minced onion
2 garlic cloves, minced

1 jalapeño pepper, minced
2 tablespoons freshly squeezed lime juice
2 tablespoons coconut milk
2 tablespoons unsalted peanut butter
2 teaspoons curry powder

Directions:

In a medium bowl, mix the pork, onion, garlic, jalapeño, lime juice, coconut milk, peanut butter, and curry powder until well combined. Set aside within 10 minutes at room temperature.

With a slotted spoon, remove the pork from the marinade. Reserve the marinade.

Thread the pork onto about 8 bamboo or metal skewers. Grill for 9 to 14 minutes, brushing once with the reserved marinade until the pork reaches at least 145°F on a meat thermometer.

Discard any remaining marinade. Serve immediately.

Nutrition:

Calories: 194
Fat: 7g
Protein: 25g
Carbohydrates: 7g
Sodium: 65mg
Fiber: 1g
Sugar: 3g

190. Pork Burgers with Red Cabbage Salad

Preparation time: 15 minutes
Cooking time: 9 minutes
Servings: 4

Ingredients:

½ cup Greek yogurt
2 tablespoons low-sodium mustard, divided
1 tablespoon lemon juice
¼ cup sliced red cabbage
¼ cup grated carrots
1-pound lean ground pork
½ teaspoon paprika
1 cup mixed baby lettuce greens
2 small tomatoes, sliced
8 small low-sodium whole-wheat sandwich buns, cut in half

Directions:

In a small bowl, combine the yogurt, 1 tablespoon mustard, lemon juice, cabbage, and carrots; mix and refrigerate.

In a medium bowl, combine the pork, remaining 1 tablespoon mustard, and paprika. Form into 8 small patties.

Put the sliders into the air fryer basket. Grill for 7 to 9 minutes, or until the sliders register 165°F as tested with a meat thermometer.

Assemble the burgers by placing some of the lettuce greens on a bun bottom. Top with a tomato slice, the -burgers, and the cabbage mixture. Add the bun top and serve immediately.

Nutrition:

Calories: 472
Fat 15g
Protein: 35g
Carbohydrates: 51g
Sodium 138mg
Sugar 8g
Fiber 8g

191. Crispy Mustard Pork Tenderloin

Preparation time: 15 minutes
Cooking time: 16 minutes
Servings: 4

Ingredients:

3 tablespoons low-sodium grainy mustard
2 teaspoons olive oil
¼ teaspoon dry mustard powder
1 (1-pound) pork tenderloin
2 slices low-sodium whole-wheat bread, crumbled
¼ cup ground walnuts
2 tablespoons cornstarch

Directions:

In a small bowl, stir the mustard, olive oil, and mustard powder. Spread this mixture over the pork.

On a plate, mix the bread crumbs, walnuts, and cornstarch. Dip the mustard-coated pork into the crumb -mixture to coat.

Air-fry the pork for 12 to 16 minutes, or until it registers at least 145°F on a meat thermometer. Slice to serve.

Nutrition:

Calories: 239
Fat: 9g
Protein: 26g
Carbohydrates: 15g
Sodium: 118mg
Fiber: 2g
Sugar: 3g

192. Espresso-Grilled Pork Tenderloin

Preparation time: 15 minutes
Cooking time: 11 minutes
Servings: 4

Ingredients:

1 tablespoon packed brown sugar
2 teaspoons espresso powder
1 teaspoon ground paprika
½ teaspoon dried marjoram
1 tablespoon honey
1 tablespoon freshly squeezed lemon juice
2 teaspoons olive oil
1 (1-pound) pork tenderloin

Directions:

Mix the brown sugar, espresso powder, paprika, and marjoram in a small bowl.

Stir in the honey, lemon juice, and olive oil until well mixed.

Spread the honey mixture over the pork and let stand for 10 minutes at room temperature.

Roast the tenderloin in the air fryer basket for 9 to 11 minutes, or until the pork registers at least 145°F on a meat thermometer. Slice the meat to serve.

Nutrition:

Calories: 177
Fat: 5g
Protein: 23g
Carbohydrates: 10g
Sodium: 61mg
Fiber: 1g
Sugar: 8g

193. Pork and Potatoes

Preparation time: 15 minutes
Cooking time: 25 minutes
Servings: 4
Ingredients:
2 cups creamer potatoes, rinsed and dried
2 teaspoons olive oil
1-pound pork tenderloin,1-inch cubes
1 onion, chopped
1 red bell pepper, chopped
2 garlic cloves, minced
½ teaspoon dried oregano
2 tablespoons low-sodium chicken broth
Directions:
Toss the potatoes and olive oil to coat in a medium bowl.
Put the potatoes in the air fryer basket—roast for 15 minutes.
In a medium metal bowl, mix the potatoes, pork, onion, red bell pepper, garlic, and oregano.
Drizzle with the chicken broth. Put the bowl in the air fryer basket.
Roast for about 10 minutes more, shaking the basket once during cooking, until the pork reaches at least 145°F on a meat thermometer and the potatoes are tender. Serve immediately.
Nutrition:
Calories: 235
Fat: 5g
Protein: 26g
Carbohydrates: 22g
Sodium: 66mg
Fiber: 3g
Sugar: 4g

194. Light Herbed Meatballs

Preparation time: 15 minutes
Cooking time: 17 minutes
Servings: 24
Ingredients:
1 medium onion, minced
2 garlic cloves, minced
1 teaspoon olive oil
1 slice low-sodium whole-wheat bread, crumbled
3 tablespoons 1 percent milk
1 teaspoon dried marjoram
1 teaspoon dried basil
1-pound 96 percent lean ground beef
Directions:
In a 6-by-2-inch pan, combine the onion, garlic, and olive oil. Air-fry for 2 to 4 minutes, or until the vegetables are crisp-tender.
Transfer the vegetables to a medium bowl, and add the bread crumbs, milk, marjoram, and basil. Mix well.
Add the ground beef. With your hands, work the mixture gently but thoroughly until combined. Form the meat mixture into about 24 (1-inch) meatballs.
Bake the meatballs, in batches, in the air fryer basket for 12 to 17 minutes, or until they reach 160°F on a meat thermometer. Serve immediately.
Nutrition:
Calories: 190
Fat: 6g
Protein: 25g
Carbohydrates: 8g
Sodium: 120mg
Fiber: 1g
Sugar: 2g

195. Brown Rice and Beef-Stuffed Bell Peppers

Preparation time: 15 minutes
Cooking time: 16 minutes
Servings: 4
Ingredients:
4 medium bell peppers, any colors, rinsed, tops removed
1 medium onion, chopped
½ cup grated carrot
2 teaspoons olive oil
2 medium beefsteak tomatoes, chopped
1 cup cooked brown rice
1 cup chopped cooked low-sodium roast beef (see Tip)
1 teaspoon dried marjoram
Directions:
Remove the stems from the bell pepper tops and chop the tops.
In a 6-by-2-inch pan, combine the chopped bell pepper tops, onion, carrot, and olive oil—Cook for 2 to 4 minutes, or until the vegetables are crisp-tender.
Transfer the vegetables to a medium bowl. Add the -tomatoes, brown rice, roast beef, and marjoram. Stir to mix.
Stuff the vegetable mixture into the bell peppers.
Place the bell peppers in the air fryer basket.
Bake for 11 to 16 minutes, or until the peppers are tender and the filling is hot. Serve immediately.
Nutrition:
Calories: 206
Fat: 6g
Protein: 18g
Carbohydrates: 20g
Sodium: 105mg
Fiber: 3g
Sugar: 5g

196. Beef and Broccoli

Preparation time: 15 minutes
Cooking time: 18 minutes
Servings: 4
Ingredients:
2 tablespoons cornstarch
½ cup low-sodium beef broth
1 teaspoon low-sodium soy sauce
12 ounces sirloin strip steak, cut into 1-inch cubes
2½ cups broccoli florets
1 onion, chopped
1 cup sliced cremini mushrooms
1 tablespoon grated fresh ginger
Brown rice, cooked (optional)
Directions:
In a medium bowl, stir the cornstarch, beef broth, and soy sauce.
Add the beef and toss to coat. Let stand for 5 minutes at room temperature.
With a slotted spoon, transfer the beef from the broth mixture into a medium metal bowl. Reserve the broth.

Add the broccoli, onion, mushrooms, and ginger to the beef. Place the bowl into the air fryer and cook for 12 to 15 minutes or until the beef reaches at least 145°F on a meat thermometer, and the vegetables are tender.

Add the reserved broth and cook for 2 to 3 minutes more, or until the sauce boils.

Serve over hot cooked brown rice.

Nutrition:

Calories: 240

Fat: 6g

Protein: 19g

Carbohydrates: 11g

Sodium: 107mg

Fiber: 2g

Sugar: 3g

197. Beef and Fruit Stir-Fry

Preparation time: 15 minutes

Cooking time: 11 minutes

Servings: 4

Ingredients:

12 ounces sirloin tip steak, thinly sliced

1 tablespoon freshly squeezed lime juice

1 cup canned mandarin orange segments, drained, liquid reserved

1 cup canned pineapple chunks, drained, liquid reserved

1 teaspoon low-sodium soy sauce

1 tablespoon cornstarch

1 teaspoon olive oil

2 scallions, white and green parts, sliced

Brown rice, cooked (optional)

Directions:

In a medium bowl, mix the steak with the lime juice. Set aside.

In a small bowl, thoroughly mix 3 tablespoons of reserved mandarin orange juice, 3 tablespoons of reserved pineapple juice, the soy sauce, and cornstarch.

Drain the beef and transfer it to a medium metal bowl, reserving the juice. Stir the reserved liquid into the mandarin-pineapple juice mixture. Set aside.

Add the olive oil and scallions to the steak. Place the metal bowl in the air fryer, cook for 3 to 4 minutes, and shake the basket once cooking.

Stir in the mandarin oranges, pineapple, and juice -mixture. Cook for 3 to 7 minutes more, or until the sauce is bubbling and the beef is tender and reaches at least 145°F on a meat thermometer.

Stir and serve over hot cooked brown rice, if desired.

Nutrition:

Calories: 212

Fat: 4g

Protein: 19g

Carbohydrates: 28g

Sodium: 105mg

Fiber: 2g

Sugar: 22g

198. Beef Risotto

Preparation time: 15 minutes

Cooking time: 24 minutes

Servings: 4

Ingredients:

2 teaspoons olive oil

1 onion, finely chopped

3 garlic cloves, minced

½ cup chopped red bell pepper

¾ cup short-grain rice

1¼ cups low-sodium beef broth

½ cup (about 3 ounces) chopped cooked roast beef (see Tip)

3 tablespoons grated Parmesan cheese

Directions:

In a 6-by-2-inch pan, combine the olive oil, onion, garlic, and red bell pepper. Place the pan in the air fryer for 2 -minutes, or until the vegetables are crisp-tender. Remove from the air fryer.

Add the rice, beef broth, and roast beef. Return the pan to the air fryer and bake for 18 to 22 minutes, stirring once during cooking, until the rice is tender and the beef reaches at least 145°F on a meat thermometer.

Remove the pan from the air fryer. Stir in the Parmesan cheese, then serve.

Nutrition:

Calories: 227

Fat: 5g

Protein: 10g

Carbohydrates: 33g

Sodium: 88mg

Fiber: 2g

Chapter 6. Snacks & Appetizers

199. Sweet Cinnamon Peaches

Preparation time: 5 minutes
Cooking time: 10 minutes
Servings: 4

Ingredients:

2 tablespoons sugar
¼ teaspoon ground cinnamon
4 peaches, cut into wedges
Cooking spray

Directions:

Grease your air fryer basket using a cooking spray.
In a large bowl, stir the sugar and cinnamon. Add the peaches to the bowl and toss to coat evenly.
Spread the coated peaches in a single layer on the basket.
Select Air Fry, set the temperature to 350ºF (180ºC), and set time to 10 minutes.
After 5 minutes, remove and flip the peaches over. Lightly mist them with cooking spray. Return until done.
Let rest for 5 minutes before serving.

Nutrition:

Calories: 80
Carbs: 20g
Fat: 0g
Protein: 0g

200. Roasted Grapes with Yogurt

Preparation time: 5 minutes
Cooking time: 10 minutes
Servings: 6

Ingredients:

2 cups seedless red grapes, rinsed and patted dry
1 tablespoon apple cider vinegar
1 tablespoon honey
1 cup low-fat Greek yogurt
2 tablespoons 2 percent milk
2 tablespoons minced fresh basil

Directions:

Spread the red grapes in the baking pan and drizzle with the cider vinegar and honey. Lightly toss to coat.
Select Roast, set temperature to 380ºF (193ºC), and set time to 10 minutes.
Whisk the yogurt and milk in a medium bowl. Gently fold in the grapes and basil.
Serve immediately.

Nutrition:

Calories: 100
Carbs: 0g
Fat: 2g
Protein: 8g

201. Garlic Edamame

Preparation time: 5 minutes
Cooking time: 9 minutes
Servings: 4

Ingredients:

1 bag frozen edamame in pods
2 tablespoon olive oil, divided
½ teaspoon garlic salt
½ teaspoon salt
¼ teaspoon freshly ground black pepper
½ teaspoon red pepper flakes (optional)

Directions:

Put the edamame in a medium bowl, then drizzle with 1 tablespoon of olive oil. Toss to coat well.
Stir the garlic salt, salt, pepper, and red pepper flakes (if desired) in a small bowl. Pour the mixture into the bowl of edamame and toss until the edamame is fully coated.
Grease your air fryer basket with the rest of the 1 tablespoon of olive oil.
Place the edamame in the greased basket.
Select Air Fry, set temperature to 375ºF (190ºC), and set time to 9 minutes.
Stir the edamame once halfway through the cooking time. Serve warm.

Nutrition:

Calories: 240
Carbs: 26g
Fat: 7g
Protein: 21g

202. Baked Sardines with Tomato Sauce

Preparation time: 10 minutes
Cooking time: 20 minutes
Servings: 4

Ingredients:

2 pounds (907 g) fresh sardines
3 tablespoons olive oil, divided
4 Roma tomatoes, peeled and chopped
1 small onion, sliced thinly
Zest of 1 orange
Sea salt
ground pepper
2 tablespoons whole-wheat bread crumbs
½ cup white wine

Directions:

Grease your baking pan using a little olive oil. Set aside.
Rinse the sardines under running water. Slit the belly, remove the spine, and butterfly the fish. Set aside.
Heat the remaining olive oil in a large skillet. Add the tomatoes, onion, orange zest, salt, and pepper to the skillet and simmer for 20 minutes, or until the mixture thickens and softens.
Put half of the sauce inside the greased pan. Arrange the sardines on top and spread the remaining half the sauce over the fish. Sprinkle with the bread crumbs and drizzle with the white wine.
Choose Convection Bake, set temperature to 425ºF (220ºC), and set time to 20 minutes.
Remove the pan from the oven, then serve immediately.

Nutrition:

Calories: 160
Carbs: 2g
Fat: 9g
Protein: 17g

203. Cheesy Baked Potatoes

Preparation time: 5 minutes
Cooking time: 20 minutes
Servings: 6

Ingredients:
12 small red potatoes
1 teaspoon kosher salt, divided
1 tablespoon extra-virgin olive oil
¼ cup grated sharp Cheddar cheese
¼ cup sour cream
2 tablespoons chopped chives
2 tablespoons grated Parmesan cheese
Directions:
Add the potatoes to a large bowl. Sprinkle with the ½ teaspoon of the salt and drizzle with the olive oil. Toss to coat. Place the potatoes in the baking pan.
Slide the baking pan into Rack Position 2, select Roast, set temperature to 375ºF (190ºC), and set time to 15 minutes.
Remove, then let the potatoes rest for 5 minutes. Halve the potatoes lengthwise. Scoop the potato flesh using a spoon into a bowl, leaving a thin shell of skin. Arrange the potato halves in the pan.
Mash the potato flesh until smooth. Mix in the remaining ½ teaspoon of the salt, Cheddar cheese, sour cream, and chives.
Transfer the filling into a pastry bag with one corner snipped off. Pipe the filling into the potato shells, mounding up slightly. Sprinkle with the Parmesan cheese.
Select Roast, temperature to 375ºF (190ºC), and set time to 5 minutes.
Let the potatoes cool slightly before serving.
Nutrition:
Calories: 135
Carbs: 22g
Fat: 4g
Protein: 4g

204. Sausage and Onion Rolls

Preparation time: 15 minutes
Cooking time: 15 minutes
Servings: 12
Ingredients:
1-pound (454 g) bulk breakfast sausage
½ cup finely chopped onion
½ cup fresh bread crumbs
½ teaspoon dried mustard
½ teaspoon dried sage
¼ teaspoon cayenne pepper
1 large egg, beaten
1 garlic clove, minced
2 sheets frozen puff pastry, thawed
All-purpose flour, for dusting
Directions:
In a medium bowl, break up the sausage. Stir in the onion, bread crumbs, mustard, sage, cayenne pepper, egg, and garlic.
Divide the sausage mixture in half and tightly wrap each half in plastic wrap. Refrigerate for 5 to 10 minutes.
Lay the pastry sheets on a lightly floured work surface. Lightly roll out the pastry to smooth out the dough.
Take out one of the sausage packages and form the sausage into a long roll. Remove the plastic wrap and place the sausage on top of the puff pastry about 1 inch from one of the long edges.
Roll the pastry around the sausage and pinch the edges of the dough together to seal. Repeat with the other pastry sheet and sausage.
Slice the logs into lengths about 1½ inches long.
Place the sausage rolls in the baking pan, cut-side down.
Choose 'Roast", temperature to 350ºF (180ºC), and set time to 15 minutes.
Let cool for 5 minutes before serving.
Nutrition:
Calories: 94
Carbs: 10g
Fat: 4g
Protein: 3g

205. Green Chiles Nachos

Preparation time: 15 minutes
Cooking time: 10 minutes
Servings: 6
Ingredients:
8 ounces (227 g) tortilla chips
3 cups shredded Monterey Jack cheese, divided
2 (7-ounce / 198-g) cans chopped green chilies, drained
1 (8-ounce / 227-g) can tomato sauce
¼ teaspoon dried oregano
¼ teaspoon granulated garlic
¼ teaspoon freshly ground black pepper
Pinch cinnamon
Pinch cayenne pepper
Directions:
Arrange the tortilla chips close together in a single layer in the baking pan. Sprinkle 1½ cups of the cheese over the chips.
Arrange the green chilies over the cheese as evenly as possible. Top with the remaining 1½ cups of the cheese.
Select "Roast," temperature to 375ºF (190ºC), and set time to 10 minutes.
Meanwhile, stir the remaining ingredients in a bowl for the sauce.
Remove from when done, then drizzle the sauce over the nachos and serve warm.
Nutrition:
Calories: 5
Carbs: 1g
Fat: 0g
Protein: 0g

206. Parmesan Cauliflower

Preparation time: 15 minutes
Cooking time: 15 minutes
Servings: 5
Ingredients:
8 cups small cauliflower florets (about 1¼ pounds / 567 g)
3 tablespoons olive oil
1 teaspoon garlic powder
½ teaspoon salt
½ teaspoon turmeric
¼ cup shredded Parmesan cheese
Directions:

In a bowl, combine the cauliflower florets, olive oil, garlic powder, salt, turmeric, and toss to coat. Transfer to the air fryer basket.
Select "Air Fry" temperature to 390ºF (199ºC), and set time to 15 minutes.
After 5 minutes, remove, then stir the cauliflower florets. Return to the oven and continue cooking.
After 6 minutes, remove and stir the cauliflower again. Return and cook again for 4 minutes. The cauliflower florets should be crisp-tender.
Sprinkle with the shredded Parmesan cheese and toss well. Serve warm.

Nutrition:
Calories: 58
Carbs: 6g
Fat: 3g
Protein: 3g

207. Cheesy Roasted Jalapeño Poppers

Preparation time: 15 minutes
Cooking time: 15 minutes
Servings: 8

Ingredients:
6 ounces (170 g) cream cheese, at room temperature
4 ounces (113 g) shredded Cheddar cheese
1 teaspoon chili powder
12 large jalapeño peppers, deseeded and sliced in half lengthwise
2 slices cooked bacon, chopped
¼ cup panko bread crumbs
1 tablespoon butter, melted

Directions:
Mix the cream cheese, Cheddar cheese, and chili powder in a medium bowl. Spoon the cheese mixture into the jalapeño halves and arrange them in the baking pan.
In a small bowl, stir the bacon, bread crumbs, and butter. Sprinkle the mixture over the jalapeño halves.
Roast, then temperature to 375ºF (190ºC) and set time to 15 minutes.
Remove, then let the poppers cool for 5 minutes before serving.

Nutrition:
Calories: 280
Carbs: 24g
Fat: 19g
Protein: 4g

208. Salty Baked Almonds

Preparation time: 5 minutes
Cooking time: 25 minutes
Servings: 4

Ingredients:
1 cup of raw almonds
1 egg white, beaten
½ teaspoon coarse sea salt

Directions:
Spread the almonds in the baking pan in an even layer.
Choose the "Convection Bake" set temperature to 350ºF (180ºC) and set time to 20 minutes.
Remove, then coat the almonds with the egg white and sprinkle with the salt. Return the pan to the oven within 5 minutes.
Cool completely before serving.

Nutrition:
Calories: 180
Carbs: 5g
Fat: 16g
Protein: 6g

209. Air Fried Lemon-Pepper Wings

Preparation time: 5 minutes
Cooking time: 24 minutes
Servings: 10

Ingredients:
2 pounds (907 g) chicken wings
4½ teaspoons salt-free lemon pepper seasoning
1½ teaspoons baking powder
1½ teaspoons kosher salt

Directions:
Toss all the fixings until well coated in a large bowl.
Put the wings in the air fryer basket, making sure they don't crowd each other too much.
Select "Air Fry" set temperature to 375ºF (190ºC) and set time to 24 minutes.
After 12 minutes, remove and turn the wings over. Return to the oven to continue cooking until done.
Let rest for 5 minutes before serving.

Nutrition:
Calories: 110
Carbs: 0g
Fat: 9g
Protein: 8g

210. Spicy and Sweet Roasted Nuts

Preparation time: 5 minutes
Cooking time: 15 minutes
Servings: 4

Ingredients:
1-pound (454 g) walnut halves and pieces
½ cup granulated sugar
3 tablespoons vegetable oil
1 teaspoon cayenne pepper
½ teaspoon fine salt

Directions:
Soak the walnuts in a large bowl with boiling water for a minute or two. Drain the walnuts.
Stir in the sugar, oil, and cayenne pepper to coat well.
Spread the walnuts in a single layer in the baking pan.
Select "Roast" set temperature to 325ºF (163ºC) and set time to 15 minutes.
After 7 or 8 minutes, remove, and stir the nuts.
Return, and check frequently.
When done, the walnuts should be dark golden brown. Sprinkle the nuts with the salt and let cool.
Serve warm.

Nutrition:
Calories: 205
Carbs: 5g
Fat: 20g
Protein: 4g

211. Paprika Deviled Eggs

Preparation time: 20 minutes
Cooking time: 16 minutes
Servings: 12

Ingredients:

3 cups ice
12 large eggs
½ cup mayonnaise
10 hamburger dill pickle chips, diced
¼ cup diced onion
2 teaspoons salt
2 teaspoons yellow mustard
1 teaspoon freshly ground black pepper
½ teaspoon paprika

Directions:

Put the ice in a large bowl, then set aside. Carefully place the eggs in the baking pan.

Set "Convection Bake," set the temperature to 250ºF (121ºC), and set time to 16 minutes.

After that, transfer the eggs to the large bowl of ice to cool.

Peel the eggs, then slice it in half lengthwise, then take out yolks into a small bowl.

Stir in the mayonnaise, pickles, onion, salt, mustard, and pepper. Mash the mixture with a fork until well combined.

Fill each egg white half with 1 to 2 teaspoons of the egg yolk mixture.

Put the paprika on top and serve immediately.

Nutrition:

Calories: 150
Carbs: 0g
Fat: 4g
Protein: 6g

212. Sausage Balls with Cheese

Preparation time: 10 minutes
Cooking time: 10 minutes
Servings: 8

Ingredients:

12 ounces (340 g) mild ground sausage
1½ cups baking mix
1 cup shredded mild Cheddar cheese
3 ounces cream cheese
1 to 2 tablespoons olive oil

Directions:

Line with parchment paper the air fryer basket. Set aside.

Mix the ground sausage, baking mix, Cheddar cheese, and cream cheese in a large bowl and stir to incorporate.

Divide the sausage mixture into 16 equal portions and roll them into 1-inch balls with your hands.

Arrange the sausage balls on the parchment, leaving space between each ball. Brush the sausage balls with olive oil.

Choose "Air Fry," set temperature to 325ºF (163ºC), and set time to 10 minutes.

Flip the balls halfway through the cooking time. Remove, and serve warm.

Nutrition:

Calories: 95
Carbs: 4g
Fat: 7g
Protein: 5g

213. Mozzarella Pepperoni Pizza Bites

Preparation time: 5 minutes
Cooking time: 12 minutes
Servings: 8

Ingredients:

1 cup finely shredded Mozzarella cheese
½ cup chopped pepperoni
¼ cup Marinara sauce
1 (8-ounce / 227-g) can crescent roll dough
All-purpose flour, for dusting

Directions:

In a small bowl, stir the cheese, pepperoni, and marinara sauce.

Lay the dough on a lightly floured work surface. Separate it into 4 rectangles. Firmly pinch the perforations together and pat the dough pieces flat.

Divide the cheese mixture evenly between the rectangles and spread it out over the dough, leaving a ¼-inch border.

Roll a rectangle up tightly, beginning with the short end. Pinch the edge down to seal the roll. Repeat with the remaining rolls.

Slice the rolls into 4 or 5, even slices. Place the slices in the baking pan, leaving a few inches between each slice.

Choose the "Roast" function, set the temperature to 350ºF (180ºC), and set time to 12 minutes. Serve.

Nutrition:

Calories: 190
Carbs: 27g
Fat: 6g
Protein: 7g

214. Air Fry Bacon

Preparation Time: 5 minutes
Cooking Time: 10 minutes
Servings: 11

Ingredients:

11 bacon, slices

Directions:

Put half of the bacon slices in the air fryer basket.

Cook at 400 F for 10 minutes.

Cook the rest of the half bacon slices using the same steps. Serve and enjoy.

Nutrition:

Calories 103
Fat 7.9 g
Carbohydrates 0.3 g
Sugar 0 g
Protein 7 g
Cholesterol 21 mg

215. Crunchy Bacon Bites

Preparation Time: 5 minutes
Cooking Time: 10 minutes
Servings: 12

Ingredients:

4 bacon strips
1/2 cup pork rinds, crushed
1/4 cup hot sauce

Directions:

Put the bacon pieces in a bowl, then put the hot sauce and toss well.

Put the crushed pork rinds and toss until bacon pieces are well coated.

Transfer bacon pieces in the air fryer basket and cook at 350 F for 10 minutes.

Serve and enjoy.
Nutrition:
Calories 112
Fat 9.7 g
Carbohydrates 0.3 g
Sugar 0.2 g
Protein 5.2 g
Cholesterol 3 mg

216. Easy Jalapeno Poppers

Preparation Time: 10 minutes
Cooking Time: 13 minutes
Servings: 5
Ingredients:
5 jalapeno peppers, slice in half and deseeded
2 tbsp salsa
4 oz goat cheese, crumbled
1/4 tsp chili powder
1/2 tsp garlic, minced
Pepper
Salt
Directions:
In a small bowl, mix cheese, salsa, chili powder, garlic, pepper, and salt.
Spoon cheese mixture into each jalapeno halves and place in the air fryer basket.
Cook jalapeno poppers at 350 F for 13 minutes.
Serve and enjoy.
Nutrition:
Calories 111
Fat 8.3 g
Carbohydrates 2.1 g
Sugar 1.2 g
Protein 7.3 g
Cholesterol 24 mg

217. Perfect Crab Dip

Preparation Time: 5 minutes
Cooking Time: 7 minutes
Servings: 4
Ingredients:
1 cup crabmeat
2 tbsp parsley, chopped
2 tbsp fresh lemon juice
2 tbsp hot sauce
1/2 cup green onion, sliced
2 cups cheese, grated
1/4 cup mayonnaise
1/4 tsp pepper
1/2 tsp salt
Directions:
In a 6-inch dish, mix crabmeat, hot sauce, cheese, mayo, pepper, and salt.
Put the dish in the air fryer basket, then cook dip at 400 F for 7 minutes.
Remove dish from air fryer.
Drizzle dip with lemon juice and garnish with parsley.
Serve and enjoy.
Nutrition:
Calories 313
Fat 23.9 g
Carbohydrates 8.8 g
Sugar 3.1 g
Protein 16.2 g
Cholesterol 67 mg

218. Spinach Dip

Preparation Time: 10 minutes
Cooking Time: 40 minutes
Servings: 8
Ingredients:
8 oz cream cheese, softened
1/4 teaspoon garlic powder
1/2 cup onion, minced
1/3 cup water chestnuts, chopped
1 cup mayonnaise
1 cup parmesan cheese, grated
1 cup frozen spinach, thawed and squeeze
1/2 teaspoon pepper
Directions:
Spray the air fryer baking dish using a cooking spray.
Put all the fixings into the bowl and mix.
Put the batter into the prepared baking dish and put it in the air fryer basket.
Cook at 300 F for 35-40 minutes. After 20 minutes of cooking, stir dip.
Serve and enjoy.
Nutrition:
Calories 220
Fat 20.5 g
Carbohydrates 9.3 g
Sugar 2.3 g
Protein 3.8 g
Cholesterol 41 mg

219. Sweet Potato Tots

Preparation Time: 10 minutes
Cooking Time: 31 minutes
Servings: 24
Ingredients:
2 sweet potatoes, peeled
1/2 teaspoon Cajun seasoning
Salt
Directions:
Put the water in pot and boil, then put the sweet potatoes. Boil for 15 minutes, then drains well.
Grate the boil sweet potatoes into a bowl.
Put the Cajun seasoning plus salt in grated sweet potatoes and mix until well combined.
Lightly spray your air fryer basket using a cooking spray.
Form a small tot of the mixture and put it in an air fryer basket.
Cook at 400 F within 8 minutes. Turn the sweet potato tots to another side and cook for 8 minutes more. Serve and enjoy.
Nutrition:
Calories 15
Fat 0 g
Carbohydrates 3.5 g
Sugar 0.1 g
Protein 0.2 g
Cholesterol 0 mg

220. Herb Zucchini Slices

Preparation Time: 10 minutes
Cooking Time: 15 minutes
Servings: 4

Ingredients:
2 zucchinis, sliced in half lengthwise
1 tbsp olive oil
4 tbsp parmesan cheese, grated
2 tbsp almond flour
1 tbsp parsley, chopped
Pepper
Salt
Directions:
Preheat the air fryer to 350 F.
In a bowl, mix cheese, parsley, oil, almond flour, pepper plus salt.
Top with cheese mixture the zucchini pieces and put in the air fryer basket.
Cook within 15 minutes at 350 F. Serve and enjoy.
Nutrition:
Calories 157
Fat 11.4 g
Carbohydrates 5.1 g
Sugar 1.7 g
Protein 11 g
Cholesterol 20 mg

221. Ranch Kale Chips

Preparation Time: 5 minutes
Cooking Time: 5 minutes
Servings: 4
Ingredients:
4 cups kale, stemmed
1 tbsp nutritional yeast flakes
2 tsp ranch seasoning
2 tbsp olive oil
1/4 tsp salt

Directions:
Mix all fixing into the large mixing bowl.
Lightly oiled your air fryer basket with cooking spray.
Add kale in air fryer basket and cook for 4-5 minutes at 370 F. Shake halfway, then serve and enjoy.
Nutrition:
Calories 102
Fat 7 g
Carbohydrates 8 g
Sugar 0 g
Protein 3 g
Cholesterol 0 mg

222. Curried Sweet Potato Fries

Preparation Time: 10 minutes
Cooking Time: 20 minutes
Servings: 3
Ingredients:
2 small sweet potatoes, peel and cut into fries' shape
1/4 tsp coriander
1/2 tsp curry powder
2 tbsp olive oil
1/4 tsp sea salt
Directions:
Put all ingredients into the large mixing bowl and toss well.
Spray air fryer basket with cooking spray.
Transfer sweet potato fries in the air fryer basket.
Cook for 20 minutes at 370 F. Shake halfway through.
Serve and enjoy.
Nutrition:
Calories 118
Fat 9 g
Carbohydrates 9 g
Sugar 2 g
Protein 1 g
Cholesterol 0 mg

223. Roasted Almonds

Preparation Time: 5 minutes
Cooking Time: 8 minutes
Servings: 8
Ingredients:
2 cups almonds
1/4 teaspoon pepper
1 teaspoon paprika
1 tablespoon garlic powder
1 tablespoon soy sauce
Directions:
Mix the pepper, paprika, garlic powder, and soy sauce in a bowl.
Add almonds and stir to coat.
Grease air fryer basket using a cooking spray.
Put the almonds into the air fryer basket and cook for 6-8 minutes at 320 F. Shake basket after every 2 minutes. Serve and enjoy.
Nutrition:
Calories 143
Fat 11.9 g
Carbohydrates 6.2 g
Sugar 1.3 g
Protein 5.4 g
Cholesterol 0 mg

224. Pepperoni Chips

Preparation Time: 2 minutes
Cooking Time: 8 minutes
Servings: 6
Ingredients:
6 oz pepperoni slices
Directions:
Place one batch of pepperoni slices in the air fryer basket. Cook for 8 minutes at 360 F.
Cook remaining pepperoni slices using the same steps. Serve and enjoy.
Nutrition:
Calories 51
Fat 1 g
Carbohydrates 2 g
Sugar 1.3 g
Protein 0 g
Cholesterol 0 mg

225. Crispy Eggplant

Preparation Time: 5 minutes
Cooking Time: 20 minutes
Servings: 4
Ingredients:
1 eggplant, cut into 1-inch pieces
1/2 tsp Italian seasoning
1 tsp paprika
1/2 tsp red pepper
1 tsp garlic powder
2 tbsp olive oil

Directions:
Toss all ingredients into the large mixing bowl.
Transfer eggplant mixture into the air fryer basket.
Cook at 375 F for 20 minutes. Shake your air fryer basket halfway through. Serve and enjoy.
Nutrition:
Calories 99
Fat 7.5 g
Carbohydrates 8.7 g
Sugar 4.5 g
Protein 1.5 g
Cholesterol 0 mg

226. Steak Nuggets

Preparation Time: 10 minutes
Cooking Time: 15 minutes
Servings: 4
Ingredients:
1 lb. beef steak, cut into chunks
1 large egg, lightly beaten
1/2 cup pork rind, crushed
1/2 cup parmesan cheese, grated
1/2 tsp salt
Directions:
Add egg in a small bowl.
In a shallow bowl, mix pork rind, cheese, plus salt.
Soak each steak chunk in egg, then coat with pork rind mixture and place on a plate. Place in the refrigerator for 30 minutes.
Lightly grease the air fryer basket using cooking spray. Preheat your air fryer at 400 F.
Put the steak nuggets in the air fryer basket, then cook for 15-18 minutes or until cooked. Shake after every 4 minutes. Serve and enjoy.
Nutrition:
Calories 609
Fat 38 g
Carbohydrates 2 g
Sugar 0.4 g
Protein 63 g
Cholesterol 195 mg

227. Cabbage Chips

Preparation Time: 10 minutes
Cooking Time: 30 minutes
Servings: 6
Ingredients:
1 large cabbage head, tear cabbage leaves into pieces
2 tbsp olive oil
1/4 cup parmesan cheese, grated
Pepper
Salt
Directions:
Preheat the air fryer to 250 F.
Add all the items into the large mixing bowl and toss well.
Grease your air fryer basket with cooking spray.
Divide cabbage in batches.
Add one cabbage chips batch in the air fryer basket and cook for 25-30 minutes at 250 F or until chips are crispy and lightly golden brown. Serve and enjoy.
Nutrition:
Calories 96
Fat 5.1 g
Carbohydrates 12.1 g
Sugar 6.7 g
Protein 3 g
Cholesterol 1 mg

228. Healthy Broccoli Tots

Preparation Time: 10 minutes
Cooking Time: 25 minutes
Servings: 4
Ingredients:
1 lb. broccoli, chopped
1/2 cup almond flour
1/4 cup ground flaxseed
1/2 teaspoon garlic powder
1 teaspoon salt
Directions:
Microwave the broccoli for 3 minutes, then transfer steamed broccoli into the food processor, then process.
Transfer it to a mixing bowl, then put the rest of the ingredients into the bowl and mix until well combined.
Spritz your air fryer basket using a cooking spray.
Form small broccoli tots and put it into the air fryer basket.
Cook the broccoli tots within 12 minutes at 375 F.
Serve and enjoy.
Nutrition:
Calories 161
Fat 9.2 g
Carbohydrates 12.8 g
Sugar 2.1 g
Protein 7.5 g
Cholesterol 0 mg

229. Classic French Fries

Preparation time: 35 minutes
Cooking time: 30 minutes
Servings: 6
Ingredients:
3 large russet potatoes
1 tablespoon canola oil
1 tablespoon extra-virgin olive oil
Salt
Pepper
Directions:
Peel the potatoes and cut lengthwise to create French fries.
Place the potatoes in a large bowl of cold water.
Allow the potatoes to soak in the water for at least 30 minutes, preferably an hour.
Spread the fries onto a baking sheet and coat them with the canola oil, olive oil, and salt and pepper to taste.
Transfer half of the fries to the air fryer basket. Cook for 10 minutes.
Shake the basket—Cook for an additional 5 minutes.
When the first half finished, remove the cooked fries, repeat steps 4 and 5 for the remaining fries.
Cool before serving.
Nutrition:
Calories: 168
Fat: 5g
Cholesterol: 0mg

Sodium: 38mg
Carbohydrates: 29g
Fiber: 4g
Protein: 3g

230. Olive Oil Sweet Potato Chips

Preparation time: 40 minutes
Cooking time: 20 minutes
Servings: 5

Ingredients:

3 sweet potatoes
2 teaspoons extra-virgin olive oil
1 teaspoon cinnamon (optional)
Salt
Pepper

Directions:

Cut the sweet potatoes crosswise into thin slices.
Put the sweet potatoes in a bowl of cold water for 30 minutes.
Drain the sweet potatoes. Dry the slices thoroughly with paper towels or napkins.
Place the sweet potatoes in another large bowl. Drizzle with the olive oil and sprinkle with the cinnamon, if using, and salt and pepper to taste. Toss to coat thoroughly.
Place the sweet potato slices in the air fryer. You may need to cook the chips in two batches—Cook the potatoes for 10 minutes.
Open and shake the basket. Cook the chips for an additional 10 minutes.
Cool before serving.

Nutrition:

Calories: 94
Fat: 2g
Cholesterol: 0mg
Sodium: 58mg
Carbohydrates: 20g
Fiber: 2g
Protein: 1g

231. Low-Carb Cheese-Stuffed Jalapeño Poppers

Preparation time: 15 minutes
Cooking time: 5 minutes
Servings: 5

Ingredients:

10 jalapeño peppers
6 ounces cream cheese
¼ cup shredded Cheddar cheese
2 tablespoons panko bread crumbs
Cooking oil

Directions:

Halve the jalapeños lengthwise. Remove the seeds and the white membrane.
Microwave the cream cheese within 15 seconds to soften.
Remove the bowl from the microwave, then put the Cheddar cheese. Mix well.
Stuff each of the jalapeño halves with the cheese mixture, then sprinkle the panko bread crumbs on top of each popper.
Place the poppers in the air fryer, spray cooking oil—Cook for 5 minutes.
Cool before serving.

Nutrition:

Calories: 156
Fat: 14g
Cholesterol: 43mg
Sodium: 874mg
Carbohydrates: 3g
Fiber: 1g
Protein: 4g

232. Vidalia Onion Blossom

Preparation time: 55 minutes
Cooking time: 25 minutes
Servings: 4

Ingredients:

1 large Vidalia onion
1½ cups all-purpose flour
1 teaspoon garlic powder
1 teaspoon paprika
Salt
Pepper
2 eggs
1 cup milk
Cooking oil

Directions:

Cut off the pointy stem end of the onion. Leave the root end intact. Peel the onion and place it cut-side down.
Starts with ½ inch from the root end, then cut down to make 4 spaced cuts. In each part, make 3 additional cuts. You should make 16 cuts in the onion.
Flip the onion over and fluff out the "petals."
Place the flour in a large bowl and season it with the garlic powder, paprika, and salt and pepper to taste.
In another large bowl, whisk the eggs. Add the milk and stir. It will form a batter.
Put the onion with the flour mixture in the bowl. Use a large spoon to cover the onion petals in flour.
Transfer the onion to the batter. Use a spoon or basting brush to cover the onion altogether.
Return the onion to the flour mixture. Cover completely.
Wrap the battered onion in foil and place in the freezer for 45 minutes.
Spatter the air fryer basket using cooking oil. Unwrap the foil covering and place the onion in the air fryer basket—Cook for 10 minutes.
Open and spray the onion with cooking oil. If areas of the onion are still white from the flour, focus the spray on these areas.
Cook again within 10 to 15 minutes, or until crisp.

Nutrition:

Calories: 253
Fat: 4g
Cholesterol: 87mg
Sodium: 101mg
Carbohydrates: 43g
Fiber: 2g
Protein: 10g

233. Spiced Nuts

Preparation time: 5 minutes
Cooking time: 15 minutes
Servings: 4

Ingredients:

½ teaspoon cinnamon
½ teaspoon stevia
Pepper
1 cup nuts (walnuts, pecans, and almonds work well)
1 egg white
Cooking oil

Directions:

In a small bowl, combine the cinnamon, stevia, and pepper to taste.
Place the nuts in another bowl with the egg white.
Add the spices to the nuts.
Spray the basket using cooking oil.
Place the nuts in the air fryer, then spray it using cooking oil—Cook for 10 minutes.
Shake the basket, then cook for an additional 3 to 4 minutes.
Serve warm.

Nutrition:

Calories: 210
Fat: 18g
Cholesterol: 0mg
Sodium: 237mg
Carbohydrates: 9g
Fiber: 3g
Protein: 7g

234. Pigs in a Blanket

Preparation time: 15 minutes
Cooking time: 20 minutes
Servings: 1

Ingredients:

1 (8-ounce) can of crescent rolls or croissant biscuit rolls
16 cocktail franks or mini smoked hot dogs
Cooking oil

Directions:

Divide the crescent roll dough into 8 triangles and place them on a flat work surface. Cut each triangle in half to make 16 triangles.
Dry the franks with a paper towel. Place 1 frank on the bottom of a triangle. It should be the widest part of the dough. Roll up the dough. Repeat for the remaining franks and triangles.
Spray your air fryer basket using cooking oil.
Place 8 pigs in a blanket in the air fryer. It is okay to stack them, but do not overcrowd the basket. Spray with cooking oil—Cook for 8 minutes.
Remove the cooked pigs in a blanket from the air fryer, then repeat step 4 for the remaining 8 pigs in a blanket. Cool before serving.

Nutrition:

Calories: 75
Fat: 5g
Cholesterol: 5mg
Sodium: 170mg
Carbohydrates: 6g
Fiber: 0g
Protein: 2g

235. Crunchy Pork Egg Rolls

Preparation time: 15 minutes
Cooking time: 15 minutes
Servings: 1

Ingredients:

Cooking oil
2 garlic cloves, minced
1 teaspoon sesame oil
¼ cup of soy sauce
2 teaspoons grated fresh ginger
12 ounces ground pork
½ cabbage, shredded (2 cups)
4 scallions, green parts (white parts optional), chopped
24 egg roll wrappers

Directions:

Spray a skillet using cooking oil, then place over medium-high heat. Add the garlic. Cook for 1 minute, until fragrant.
Add the ground pork to the skillet. Using a spoon, break the pork into smaller chunks.
Mix the sesame oil, soy sauce, and ginger in a small bowl.
Add the sauce to the skillet. Stir to combine. Continue cooking for 5 minutes, until the pork is browned.
When the pork has browned, add the cabbage and scallions. Mix well.
Transfer the pork mixture to a large bowl.
Lay the egg roll wrappers on a flat surface. Dip a basting brush in water and glaze each of the egg roll wrappers along the edges with the wet brush.
Stack 2 egg roll wrappers. Scoop 1 to 2 tablespoons of the pork mixture onto the center.
Roll one long side of the wrappers up over the filling. Press firmly on the area with the filling, tucking it in lightly to secure it in place. Fold in the left and right sides.
Continue rolling to close. Use the basting brush to wet the seam and seal the egg roll.
Place the egg rolls in the basket of the air fryer. It is okay to stack them. Then, spray cooking oil—Cook for 8 minutes.
Flip the egg rolls. Cook for an additional 4 minutes.
Cool before serving.

Nutrition:

Calories: 244
Fat: 4g
Cholesterol: 27mg
Sodium: 683mg
Carbohydrates: 39g
Fiber: 2g
Protein: 12g

236. Spinach and Artichoke Dip Wontons

Preparation time: 15 minutes
Cooking time: 40 minutes
Servings: 10

Ingredients:

6 ounces cream cheese
¼ cup sour cream
¼ cup shredded Parmesan cheese
¼ cup shredded mozzarella cheese
5 ounces frozen chopped spinach
6 ounces marinated artichoke hearts, drained
2 garlic cloves, chopped
Salt
Pepper
20 wonton wrappers
Cooking oil

Directions:

Microwave the cream cheese within 20 seconds to soften.

Mix the cream cheese, sour cream, Parmesan, mozzarella, spinach, artichoke hearts, garlic, salt, and pepper to taste in a medium bowl. Stir to mix well.

Arrange the wonton wrappers on your cutting board. Scoop 1½ teaspoons of the artichoke mixture onto each wrapper. Be careful not to overfill.

Fold each wrapper diagonally to form a triangle. Bring the two bottom corners up toward each other. Do not close the wrapper yet. Bring up the two open sides and push out any air. Squeeze the open edges together to seal.

Place the wontons in the air fryer basket and cook in batches or stack. Spray the wontons with cooking oil—Cook for 10 minutes.

Remove the basket and flip the wontons. Return it and cook for an additional 5 to 8 minutes, until the wontons have reached your desired level of golden-brown crispiness.

Cool before serving.

Nutrition:

Calories: 166
Fat: 7g
Cholesterol: 14mg
Sodium: 345mg
Carbohydrates: 21g
Fiber: 1g
Protein: 5g

237. Loaded Disco Fries

Preparation time: 15 minutes
Cooking time: 25 minutes
Servings: 5

Ingredients:

1 (28-ounce) bag frozen steak fries
Cooking oil
Salt
Pepper
½ cup beef gravy
1 cup shredded mozzarella cheese
2 scallions, green parts only, chopped

Directions:

Place the frozen steak fries in the air fryer. Cook for 10 minutes.

Open and shake, then spray the fries with cooking oil. Sprinkle with salt and pepper to taste—Cook for an additional 8 minutes.

Pour the beef gravy into a medium, microwave-safe bowl—microwave for 30 seconds, or until the gravy is warm.

Sprinkle the fries with the cheese—Cook for an additional 2 minutes until the cheese is melted.

Transfer the fries to a serving dish. Drizzle the fries with gravy and sprinkle the scallions on top for a green garnish. Serve.

Nutrition:

Calories: 291
Fat: 11g
Cholesterol: 18mg
Sodium: 774mg
Carbohydrates: 39g
Fiber: 3g
Protein: 1g

238. Fried Olives

Preparation time: 15 minutes
Cooking time: 10 minutes
Servings: 4

Ingredients:

1 (5½-ounce) jar pitted green olives
½ cup all-purpose flour
Salt
Pepper
½ cup bread crumbs
1 egg
Cooking oil

Directions:

Pat dry using a paper cloth the olives from the jar.

Mix the flour with salt and pepper to taste in a small bowl. Place the bread crumbs in another small bowl. In a third small bowl, beat the egg.

Grease the basket using cooking oil.

Dip the olives in the flour, then the egg, and then the bread crumbs.

Place the breaded olives in the air fryer. It is okay to stack them. Spray the olives with cooking oil—Cook for 6 minutes.

Flip the olives. Cook again within 2 minutes, or until brown and crisp.

Cool before serving.

Nutrition:

Calories: 165
Fat: 5g
Cholesterol: 41mg
Sodium: 828mg
Carbohydrates: 24g
Fiber: 4g
Protein: 5g

239. Potato Skin Bites

Preparation time: 15 minutes
Cooking time: 20 minutes
Servings: 25

Ingredients:

4 slices bacon
4 large russet potatoes
1 tablespoon extra-virgin olive oil
1 teaspoon paprika
Salt
Pepper
1 cup shredded Cheddar cheese
2 teaspoons chopped chives
2 teaspoons chopped scallions, green parts (white parts optional)

Directions:

Cook all the bacon in a skillet, for about 5 to 7 minutes, flipping to evenly crisp. Drain on paper towels, crumble, and set aside.

Cut the potatoes into ½-inch-thick rounds. Place the potato rounds in a large bowl with the olive oil and paprika, and season with salt and pepper to taste. Toss to coat thoroughly.

Put all the potatoes in your air fryer basket. It is okay to stack them, but do not overcrowd the basket. You may need to cook the potatoes in two batches—Cook for 10 minutes.

Open, then shake it. Cook for an additional 5 to 8 minutes, until the potato skin bites, are soft in the middle and crisp along the edges.
Transfer the potato skin bites to a serving dish. Top with the shredded cheese, crumbled bacon, chives, and scallions. Serve.

Nutrition:
Calories: 81
Fat: 3g
Cholesterol: 8mg
Sodium: 110mg
Carbohydrates: 9g
Fiber: 2g
Protein: 3g

240. Jalapeno & Cheddar Cornbread Muffins

Preparation time: 15 minutes
Cooking time: 30 minutes
Servings: 8

Ingredients:
½ cup yellow cornmeal
¼ cup all-purpose flour
¼ cup of sugar
1 tsp baking powder
¼ tsp baking soda
½ tsp salt
½ cup buttermilk
½ can creamed corn
1 egg, beaten
2 tbsp unsalted butter, melted
1 cup shredded sharp cheddar cheese
1 fresh jalapeño pepper,
Cooking spray

Directions:
Mix the sugar, baking powder, baking soda, cornmeal, flour plus salt.
Put in the buttermilk, creamed corn, egg, melted butter, cheddar cheese, plus minced jalapeño.
Grease the muffin pan with cooking spray.
Split the batter between 8 of the 12 muffin cups and set aside.
Insert the wire rack at a low position in the Air Fryer Oven. Select "Bake" set the timer to 30 minutes.
Remove, then cool it down for 10 minutes before serving.

Nutrition:
Calories 192
Fat 8.8g
Carbs 21.9g
Protein 6.3g

241. Roasted Garlic

Preparation time: 15 minutes
Cooking time: 30 minutes
Servings: 10

Ingredients:
3 whole garlic bulbs, halved
3 tablespoons olive oil
¼ teaspoon kosher salt

Directions:
Choose the "Bake" function on the Air Fryer Oven, set time to 30 minutes to preheat.
Rub and drizzle garlic halves with olive oil plus salt.
Arrange the food tray with parchment paper, then place garlic bulb halves face down onto the food tray.
Insert the food tray at a low position in the preheated air fryer toaster oven.
Turn the garlic halves face up after cooking for 20 minutes.
Remove garlic halves when done, serve as a side, or make it into a paste to spread with butter over Toast.

Nutrition:
Calories 39
Fat 4.2g
Carbs 0.2g
Protein 0.3g

242. Chili Beef Nachos

Preparation time: 15 minutes
Cooking time: 5 minutes
Servings: 3

Ingredients:
1 can chili
½ tsp cumin
¼ tsp oregano
¼ tsp taco seasoning
black pepper
1 bag tortilla chips
1 bag Mexican blend shredded cheese
Mexican crema, for drizzling

Directions:
Microwave the chili, cumin, oregano, taco seasoning, and black pepper within 1 minute, then set aside.
Insert the wire rack at the top position in the Air Fryer Oven. Select the Broil function, set the timer to 5 minutes.
Place half of the tortilla chips in the broiler pan lined with foil, top them with half the chili, and then half the cheese. Repeat this process to add a second layer of nachos.
Put the broiler pan on top of the wire rack in the preheated air fryer toaster oven and press Start/Cancel.
Remove when done, drizzle with Mexican crema, then serve.

Nutrition:
Calories 466
Fat 32.7g
Carbs 30g
Protein 13g

243. Salted Maple Pecan Granola

Preparation time: 15 minutes
Cooking time: 40 minutes
Servings: 4

Ingredients:
2 cups old fashioned oats
1 cup pecans, chopped
2 tbsp dark brown sugar, packed
¾ tsp kosher salt
1 tsp ground cinnamon
¼ tsp ground nutmeg
¼ cup coconut oil, melted
½ cup maple syrup
½ tsp maple extract

Directions:

Mix all fixings in a large bowl, then line the food tray with parchment paper and spread the granola evenly on top. Set aside.
Select the Bake on the Air Fryer Oven, set time to 40 minutes.
Stir the granola every 10 minutes to ensure even baking.
Remove granola when done and allow to cool for 1 hour.
Break granola into chunks and enjoy immediately, or store in an airtight container afterward.

Nutrition:
Calories 577
Fat 21.4g
Carbs 85.6g
Protein 10.4g

244. Bacon-Wrapped Hot Dogs

Preparation time: 15 minutes
Cooking time: 20 minutes
Servings: 4

Ingredients:
4 strips thick-cut bacon
4 beef hot dogs
4 hot dog buns, slightly toasted

Directions:
Cover 1 piece of bacon around each beef hot dog, allowing the bacon's edges to overlap slightly. Set aside.
Select "Broil" on the Air Fryer Oven, set time to 20 minutes.
Line the food tray with foil, then set the wire rack on top of the food tray.
Place the bacon-wrapped hot dogs on the wire rack, then insert the rack and food tray at the top position in the preheated air fryer oven.
Flip the hot dogs halfway through cooking.
Remove and place each hot dog in a hot dog bun.
Serve with your choice of toppings.

Nutrition:
Calories 265
Fat 13g
Carbs 24g
Protein 13g

245. Double-Baked Stuffed Potato

Preparation time: 15 minutes
Cooking time: 75 minutes
Servings: 2

Ingredients:
2 large russet potatoes
2 tablespoons butter
½ cup heavy whipping cream
¼ teaspoon kosher salt
¼ cup sour cream
¼ cup shredded cheddar cheese
2 slices cooked bacon, cut into bits
1 green onion, sliced

Directions:
Select Bake, set time to 1 hour, and temperature to 350°F.
Put the potatoes on the wire rack and insert them at mid-position in the preheated air fryer oven.
Remove, then cool it for 5 minutes.
Scoop out the insides of the potatoes into a large bowl.
Put the butter, heavy whipping cream, and kosher salt to the bowl and mash it.
Put the mashed potatoes into the potato skins and put back in the air fryer toaster oven.
Bake again, set time to 15 minutes and temperature to 350°F, then press Start/Cancel twice to forgo preheating.
Remove potatoes and garnish with sour cream, cheddar cheese, bacon bits, and green onion.

Nutrition:
Calories 694
Fat 41.7g
Carbs 61.1g
Protein 18.6g

246. Garlic Bread

Preparation time: 15 minutes
Cooking time: 75 minutes
Servings: 2

Ingredients:
Two 6-inch baguettes halved lengthwise
3 tablespoons unsalted butter, melted
3 cloves garlic, minced
¼ teaspoon salt
1 teaspoon dried parsley

Directions:
Mix melted butter, minced garlic, salt, and parsley.
Brush mixture over each baguette half.
Place baguettes on the Air Fryer Oven's wire rack and insert it at mid position.
Select the Toast, set to darkness level 6, and press Start/Cancel.
Serve immediately.

Nutrition:
Calories 271
Fat 17.7g
Carbs 23.5g
Protein 4.5g

247. Sweet & Spicy Korean Chicken Wings

Preparation time: 15 minutes
Cooking time: 35 minutes
Servings: 4

Ingredients:
2 pounds of chicken wings
2 tablespoons gochujang paste
2 tablespoons sambal chili paste
½ cup of water
2 tablespoons rice vinegar
1 teaspoon sesame oil
1 tablespoon fish sauce
2 tablespoons dark brown sugar
1 tablespoon ginger, grated
¼ teaspoon salt
1 tablespoon sesame seeds
1 green onion, sliced, for garnish

Directions:
Select the Air Fry, set time to 35 minutes.
Put the chicken wings into your fry basket, then insert the basket at mid-position.

Mix the water, rice vinegar, sesame oil, fish sauce, gochujang paste, sambal chili paste, dark brown sugar, ginger, and salt in a small saucepan and mix. Cook Set the saucepan over medium-high heat for 8 minutes, or until reduced by half.
Take out chicken wings when done, and put in a separate bowl.
Pour the sauce over the chicken wings, then toss to make sure they're well coated.
Sprinkle sesame seeds and sliced green onions to garnish, then serve.
Nutrition:
Calories 483
Fat 19g
Carbs 11g
Protein 67g

248. Honey Mustard Chicken Legs

Preparation time: 15 minutes
Cooking time: 35 minutes
Servings: 3
Ingredients:
6 chicken legs
1 lemon, juiced
2 tbsp stone-ground mustard
2 tbsp honey
¼ tsp kosher salt
¼ tsp black pepper
Directions:
Dip the chicken legs in lemon juice for 15 minutes.
Choose the "Air Fry," set time to 30 minutes, and temperature to 400°F.
Mix the mustard plus honey in a small bowl, then set aside.
Put salt plus pepper on each side of the chicken legs.
Put the chicken legs in the fry basket, at mid-position in the preheated air fryer toaster oven.
Scoop half of the honey mustard batter over the chicken legs. Put the rest of the honey mustard aside.
Select the Air Fry again within 5 minutes at 400°F.
Let the chicken legs rest for 5 minutes when done, then serve with the remaining honey mustard sauce.
Nutrition:
Calories 497
Fat 29g
Carbs 16g
Protein 43g

249. Margherita Pizza

Preparation time: 15 minutes
Cooking time: 15 minutes
Servings: 6
Ingredients:
12 ounces pizza dough
2 tablespoons olive oil
¼ cup pizza sauce or tomato sauce
3 ounces low-moisture mozzarella cheese
2 tablespoons grated Parmigiano Reggiano
1 teaspoon red pepper flakes
2 sprigs basil, for garnish
Directions:
Dust flour onto your clean work surface and form the dough into a ball. Put a damp cloth over the dough and let it rest for 1 hour.
Insert wire rack at mid-position in the Air Fryer Oven. Select the Pizza function.
Shape the dough into a circle 12 inches in diameter. Put the dough onto a pizza pan.
Drizzle the olive oil onto the pizza dough evenly, making sure to brush the edges.
Spread pizza sauce evenly onto the dough, leaving a ½-inch border.
Sprinkle the mozzarella, Parmigiano Reggiano, and red pepper flakes evenly onto the pizza.
Place the pizza on top of the wire rack in the air fryer oven, select start.
Remove pizza when done. Garnish with fresh basil leaves, then serve.
Nutrition:
Calories 327
Fat 23g
Carbs 25g
Protein 5g

250. Pepperoni Pizza

Preparation time: 15 minutes
Cooking time: 15 minutes
Servings: 4
Ingredients:
12 ounces pizza dough
2 tablespoons olive oil
¼ cup tomato sauce
3 ounces low-moisture mozzarella
2 tablespoons Parmesan, grated
¼ teaspoon kosher salt
2 ounces pepperoni, sliced
Directions:
Dust the flour onto the clean work surface and form the pizza dough into a ball. Put a wet cloth on the dough, then rest it for 1 hour.
Punch down the dough, then shape or roll the dough into a thin circle up to 12 inches in diameter.
Transfer it onto a pizza pan.
Spread the olive oil onto it evenly. Spread tomato sauce evenly onto the dough, leaving a ½-inch border.
Position the wire rack at mid-position in the Air Fryer Oven. Select "Pizza", set timer to 15 minutes.
Sprinkle mozzarella, Parmesan, and salt evenly onto the pizza. Top with pepperoni.
Put the pizza pan over the rack in the preheated air fryer toaster oven. Serve.
Nutrition:
Calories 643
Fat 47g
Carbs 38g
Protein 17g

251. Rotisserie Chicken

Preparation time: 15 minutes
Cooking time: 70 minutes
Servings: 5
Ingredients:
1 whole chicken (5 pounds)
1-gallon water
¾ cup kosher salt
3 tbsp black pepper
2 bay leaves
Directions:

Whisk the water, salt, black pepper, plus bay leaves for the brine. Soak the chicken in the brine and let it sit for 1 hour.
Pat chicken dry, then truss with butcher's twine to ensure the wings and legs are held together.
Insert the rotisserie shaft through the chicken, securing the chicken between the forks. Place the shaft into the designated ports in the Air Fryer Oven.
Select the Rotisserie function, set time to 1 hour 10 minutes, and temperature to 380°F. Put the convection fan on high speed for better crispness.
Remove rotisserie chicken with the rotisserie handle when done. Carve the chicken into desired portions, then serve.
Nutrition:
Calories 82
Fat 2.8g
Carbs 3.3g
Protein 10.8g

252. Bow Tie Pasta Chips

Preparation Time: 10 minutes
Cooking Time: 10 minutes
Servings: 6
Ingredients:
2 cups white bow tie pasta
1 tablespoon olive oil
1 tablespoon nutritional yeast
1½ teaspoons Italian seasoning blend
½ teaspoon salt
Directions:
Cook the pasta for half the time base on the package.
Mix the cooked pasta with olive oil, nutritional yeast, Italian seasoning, and salt.
Put half of the batter in your air fryer basket.
Cook at 390 F within 5 minutes. Shake the basket and cook 3 to 5 minutes more or until crunchy.
Nutrition:
Calories: 408
Fat: 23.1g
Carbohydrates: 52.6g
Sugar: 0g
Protein: 14.6g
Sodium: 688mg

253. Stuffed Mushrooms with Sour Cream

Preparation Time: 15 minutes
Cooking Time: 8 minutes
Servings: 12
Ingredients:
¼ orange bell pepper, diced
¾ cup Cheddar cheese, shredded
12 mushrooms caps, stems diced
½ onion, diced
½ small carrot, diced
¼ cup sour cream
Directions:
Preheat the Air fryer to 350-degree F and grease a baking tray.
Place mushroom stems, onion, orange bell pepper, and carrot over medium heat in a skillet.
Cook within 5 minutes until softened, then stir in ½ cup Cheddar cheese and sour cream.
Stuff this mixture in the mushroom caps and arrange them on the baking tray.
Top with the rest of the cheese and place the baking tray in the Air fryer basket.
Cook for about 8 minutes until cheese is melted and serve warm.
Nutrition:
Calories: 43
Fat: 3.1g
Carbohydrates: 1.7g
Sugar: 1g
Protein: 2.4g
Sodium: 55mg

254. Crispy Shrimps

Preparation Time: 15 minutes
Cooking Time: 8 minutes
Servings: 2
Ingredients:
1 egg
¼ pound nacho chips, crushed
10 shrimps, peeled and deveined
1 tablespoon olive oil
Salt and black pepper, to taste
Directions:
Preheat the Air fryer to 3650F and grease an Air fryer basket.
Beat the egg in a bowl.
Place the nacho chips in another shallow dish.
Rub the shrimps with salt plus black pepper, coat into the egg, and roll into nacho chips.
Place the coated shrimps into the Air fryer basket and cook for about 8 minutes.
Dish out and serve warm.
Nutrition:
Calories: 514
Fat: 25.8g
Carbohydrates: 36.9g
Sugar: 2.3g
Protein: 32.5g
Sodium: 648mg

255. Sunflower Seeds Bread

Preparation Time: 15 minutes
Cooking Time: 18 minutes
Servings: 4
Ingredients:
2/3 cup whole wheat flour
2/3 cup plain flour
1/3 cup sunflower seeds
1 cup lukewarm water
½ sachet instant yeast
1 teaspoon salt
Directions:
Preheat the Air fryer to 390-degree F and grease a cake pan.
Mix the flours, sunflower seeds, yeast, and salt in a bowl.
Put the water slowly, then knead for about 5 minutes until a dough is formed.
Wrap the dough using a plastic wrap, then keep in a warm place for about half an hour.
Arrange the dough into a cake pan and transfer into an air fryer basket.

Cook for about 18 minutes and dish out to serve warm.

Nutrition:

Calories: 156
Fat: 2.4g
Carbohydrates: 28.5g
Sugar: 0.5g
Protein: 4.6g
Sodium: 582mg

256. Air Fried Chicken Tenders

Preparation Time: 15 minutes
Cooking Time: 10 minutes
Servings: 4

Ingredients:

12 oz chicken breasts, cut into tenders
1 egg white
1/8 cup flour
½ cup panko bread crumbs
Salt and black pepper, to taste

Directions:

Preheat the Air fryer to 350-degree F and grease an Air fryer basket.
Rub the chicken tenders with salt plus black pepper.
Coat the chicken tenders with flour, then dip in egg whites and then dredge in the panko bread crumbs.
Arrange in the Air fryer basket and cook for about 10 minutes.
Dish out in a platter and serve warm.

Nutrition:

Calories: 220
Fat: 17.1g
Carbohydrates: 6g
Sugar: 3.5g
Protein: 12.8g
Sodium: 332mg

257. Air Fryer Plantains

Preparation Time: 10 minutes
Cooking Time: 10 minutes
Servings: 4

Ingredients:

2 ripe plantains
2 teaspoons avocado oil
1/8 teaspoon salt

Directions:

Preheat the Air fryer to 400-degree F and grease an Air fryer basket.
Mix the plantains with avocado oil and salt in a bowl.
Arrange the coated plantains in the Air fryer basket and cook for about 10 minutes.
Dish out in a bowl and serve immediately.

Nutrition:

Calories: 112
Fat: 0.6g
Carbohydrates: 28.7g
Sugar: 13.4g
Protein: 1.2g
Sodium: 77mg

258. Pita Bread Cheese Pizza

Preparation Time: 10 minutes
Cooking Time: 6 minutes
Servings: 4

Ingredients:

1 pita bread
¼ cup Mozzarella cheese
7 slices pepperoni
¼ cup sausage
1 tablespoon yellow onion, sliced thinly
1 tablespoon pizza sauce
1 drizzle extra-virgin olive oil
½ teaspoon fresh garlic, minced

Directions:

Preheat the Air fryer to 350-degree F and grease an Air fryer basket.
Spread pizza sauce on the pita bread and add sausages, pepperoni, onions, garlic, and cheese.
Drizzle with olive oil and place it in the air fryer basket.
Cook for about 6 minutes and dish out to serve warm.

Nutrition:

Calories: 56
Fat: 3.6g
Carbohydrates: 6.7g
Sugar: 3.6g
Protein: 0.3g
Sodium: 0mg

259. Buttered Dinner Rolls

Preparation Time: 15 minutes
Cooking Time: 30 minutes
Servings: 12

Ingredients:

1 cup milk
3 cups plain flour
7½ tablespoons unsalted butter
1 tablespoon coconut oil
1 tablespoon olive oil
1 teaspoon yeast
Salt and black pepper, to taste

Directions:

Preheat the Air fryer to 360-degree F and grease an Air fryer basket.
Put olive oil, milk, and coconut oil in a pan and cook for about 3 minutes.
Remove from the heat and mix well.
Mix plain flour, yeast, butter, salt, and black pepper in a large bowl.
Knead well for about 5 minutes until a dough is formed.
Wrap the dough using a wet cloth and keep aside for about 5 minutes in a warm place.
Knead the dough within 5 minutes again with your hands.
Cover the dough again with a moist cloth and keep aside for about 30 minutes in a warm place.
Divide the dough into 12 equal pieces and roll each into a ball.
Arrange 6 balls into the Air fryer basket in a single layer and cook for about 15 minutes.
Repeat with the remaining balls and serve warm.

Nutrition:

Calories: 208
Fat: 10.3g
Carbohydrates: 25g
Sugar: 1g
Protein: 4.1g

Sodium: 73mg

260. Croissant Rolls

Preparation Time: 10 minutes
Cooking Time: 6 minutes
Servings: 8

Ingredients:

8-ounces croissant rolls
4 tablespoons butter, melted
1 tablespoon olive oil

Directions:

Preheat the Air fryer to 320-degree F and grease an Air fryer basket with olive oil.
Coat the croissant rolls with butter and arrange into the Air fryer basket.
Cook for about 6 minutes, flipping once in between.
Dish out in a platter and serve hot.

Nutrition:

Calories: 167
Fat: 12.6g
Carbohydrates: 11.1g
Sugar: 3g
Protein: 2.1g
Sodium: 223mg

261. Healthy Veggie Lasagna

Preparation Time: 15 minutes
Cooking Time: 1 hour
Servings: 4

Ingredients:

1½ pounds pumpkin, peeled and chopped finely
¾ pound tomatoes, cubed
1-pound cooked beets, sliced thinly
½ pound fresh lasagna sheets
¼ cup Parmesan cheese, grated
2 tablespoons sunflower oil

Directions:

Preheat the Air fryer to 300-degree F and lightly grease a baking dish.
Put pumpkin and 1 tablespoon sunflower oil in a skillet and cook for about 10 minutes.
Put the pumpkin mixture and tomatoes in a blender and pulse until smooth.
Return to the skillet and cook on low heat for about 5 minutes.
Transfer the pumpkin puree into the baking dish and layer with lasagna sheets.
Top with the beet slices and cheese and place in the air fryer.
Cook for about 45 minutes and dish out to serve warm.

Nutrition:

Calories: 368
Fats: 10.3g
Carbohydrates: 59.8g
Sugar: 16.9g
Proteins: 13.4g
Sodium: 165mg

262. Portabella Pizza Treat

Preparation Time: 10 minutes
Cooking Time: 6 minutes
Servings: 2

Ingredients:

2 Portabella caps, stemmed
2 tablespoons canned tomatoes with basil
2 tablespoons mozzarella cheese, shredded
4 pepperoni slices
2 tablespoons Parmesan cheese, grated freshly
2 tablespoon olive oil
1/8 teaspoon dried Italian seasonings
Salt, to taste
1 teaspoon red pepper flakes, crushed

Directions:

Preheat the Air fryer to 320-degree F and grease an Air fryer basket.
Drizzle the olive oil on each sides of portabella cap and season salt, red pepper flakes, and Italian seasonings.
Top the canned tomatoes on the mushrooms, followed by mozzarella cheese.
Place portabella caps in the Air fryer basket and cook for about 2 minutes.
Top with pepperoni slices and cook for about 4 minutes.
Sprinkle with Parmesan cheese and dish out to serve warm.

Nutrition:

Calories: 242
Fat: 21.8g
Carbohydrates: 5.8g
Sugar: 2g
Protein: 8.8g
Sodium: 350mg

263. Heirloom Tomato Sandwiches with Pesto

Preparation Time: 20 minutes
Cooking Time: 16 minutes
Servings: 2

Ingredients:

3 tablespoons pine nuts
½ cup fresh basil, chopped
½ cup fresh parsley, chopped
2 heirloom tomatoes, cut into ½ inch thick slices
8-ounce feta cheese, cut into ½ inch thick slices
½ cup plus 2 tablespoons olive oil, divided
Salt, to taste
1 garlic clove, chopped

Directions:

Preheat the Air fryer to 390-degree F and grease an Air fryer basket.
Mix 1 tablespoon of olive oil, pine nuts, and a pinch of salt in a bowl.
Place pine nuts in the air fryer and cook for about 2 minutes.
Put the pine nuts, remaining oil, fresh basil, fresh parsley, garlic, salt, and pulse until combined.
Dish out the pesto in a bowl, cover, and refrigerate.
Spread 1 tablespoon of pesto on each tomato slice and top with a feta slice and onion.
Drizzle with olive oil and arrange the prepared tomato slices in the Air fryer basket.
Cook for about 14 minutes and serve with the remaining pesto.

Nutrition:

Calories: 559
Fat: 55.7g

Carbohydrates: 8g
Sugar: 2.6g
Protein: 11.8g
Sodium: 787mg

264. Cheese Stuffed Tomatoes

Preparation Time: 15 minutes
Cooking Time: 15 minutes
Servings: 2

Ingredients:

2 large tomatoes, sliced in half and pulp scooped out
½ cup broccoli, finely chopped
½ cup cheddar cheese, shredded
1 tablespoon unsalted butter, melted
½ teaspoon dried thyme, crushed

Directions:

Preheat the Air fryer to 355-degree F and grease an Air fryer basket.
Mix broccoli and cheese in a bowl.
Stuff the broccoli mixture in each tomato.
Arrange the stuffed tomatoes into the Air fryer basket and drizzle evenly with butter.
Cook for about 15 minutes and dish out in a serving platter.
Garnish with thyme and serve warm.

Nutrition:

Calories: 206
Fat: 15.6g
Carbohydrates: 9.1g
Sugar: 5.3g
Protein: 9.4g
Sodium: 233mg

265. Hummus Mushroom Pizza

Preparation Time: 20 minutes
Cooking Time: 6 minutes
Servings: 4

Ingredients:

4 Portobello mushroom caps, stemmed and gills removed
3 ounces zucchini, shredded
2 tablespoons sweet red pepper, seeded and chopped
4 Kalamata olives, sliced
½ cup hummus
1 tablespoon balsamic vinegar
Salt and black pepper, to taste
4 tablespoons pasta sauce
1 garlic clove, minced
1 teaspoon dried basil

Directions:

Preheat the Air fryer to 330-degree F and grease an Air fryer basket.
Coat both sides of all Portobello mushroom cap with vinegar.
Season the inside of each mushroom cap with salt and black pepper.
Divide pasta sauce and garlic inside each mushroom.
Arrange mushroom caps into the Air fryer basket and cook for about 3 minutes.
Remove from the Air fryer and top zucchini, red peppers, and olives on each mushroom cap.
Season with basil, salt, and black pepper and transfer into the Air fryer basket.
Cook for about 3 more minutes and dish out in a serving platter.
Spread hummus on each mushroom pizza and serve.

Nutrition:

Calories: 115
Fat: 4.1g
Carbohydrates: 15.4g
Sugar: 4.8g
Protein: 6.7g
Sodium: 264mg

266. Rice Flour Crusted Tofu

Preparation Time: 15 minutes
Cooking Time: 28 minutes
Servings: 3

Ingredients:

1 block firm tofu, pressed and cubed into ½-inch size
2 tablespoons cornstarch
¼ cup of rice flour
Salt and ground black pepper, as required
2 tablespoons olive oil

Directions:

Preheat the Air fryer to 360-degree F and grease an Air fryer basket.
Mix the cornstarch, rice flour, salt, and black pepper in a bowl.
Coat the tofu with flour mixture evenly and drizzle with olive oil.
Arrange the tofu cubes into the Air fryer basket and cook for about 28 minutes.
Dish out the tofu in a serving platter and serve warm.

Nutrition:

Calories: 241
Fat: 15g
Carbohydrates: 17.7g
Sugar: 0.8g
Protein: 11.6g
Sodium: 67mg

Chapter 7. Fish & Seafood

267. Sole and Cauliflower Fritters

Preparation time: 5 minutes
Cooking time: 24 minutes
Servings: 2
Ingredients:
½ pound (227 g) sole fillets
½ pound (227 g) mashed cauliflower
½ cup red onion, chopped
1 bell pepper, finely chopped
1 egg, beaten
2 garlic cloves, minced
2 tablespoons fresh parsley, chopped
1 tablespoon olive oil
1 tablespoon coconut aminos
½ teaspoon scotch bonnet pepper, minced
½ teaspoon paprika
Salt and white pepper, to taste
Cooking spray
Directions:
Grease the air fry basket with cooking spray. Place the sole fillets in the basket.
Select Air Fry, Convection, set temperature to 395ºF (202ºC), and set time to 10 minutes.
Flip the fillets halfway through.
When done, transfer the fish fillets to a large bowl. Mash the fillets into flakes. Put the rest of the fixings and stir to combine.
Make the fritters: Scoop out 2 tablespoons of the fish mixture and shape into a patty about ½ inch thick with your hands, then place the patties in the air fry basket.
Set temperature to 380ºF (193ºC), and set time to 14 minutes.
Flip the patties halfway through.
Remove the basket from the oven and cool for 5 minutes before serving.
Nutrition:
Calories: 139
Carbs: 14g
Fat: 12g
Protein: 10g

268. Cheesy Tuna Patties

Preparation time: 5 minutes
Cooking time: 18 minutes
Servings: 4
Ingredients:
Tuna Patties:
1 pound (454 g) canned tuna, drained
1 egg, whisked
2 tablespoons shallots, minced
1 garlic clove, minced
1 cup grated Romano cheese
Sea salt
ground black pepper
1 tablespoon sesame oil
Cheese Sauce:
1 tablespoon butter
1 cup beer
2 tablespoons grated Colby cheese
Directions:
Mix the canned tuna, whisked egg, shallots, garlic, cheese, salt, and pepper in a large bowl and stir to incorporate.
Split the tuna mixture into four equal portions and form each portion into a patty with your hands.
Refrigerate the patties for 2 hours.
When ready, brush both sides of each patty with sesame oil, then place it in the air fry basket.
Set temperature to 360ºF (182ºC), and set time to 14 minutes.
Turn over the patties halfway through the cooking time.
Meanwhile, dissolve the butter in a saucepan over medium heat.
Pour in the beer and whisk constantly, or until it begins to bubble. Add the grated Colby cheese and mix well. Continue cooking for 3 to 4 minutes, or until the cheese melts. Remove from the heat.
Remove the patties from the oven to a plate. Drizzle them with the cheese sauce and serve immediately.
Nutrition:
Calories: 210
Carbs: 8g
Fat: 4g
Protein: 16g

269. Golden Beer-Battered Cod

Preparation time: 5 minutes
Cooking time: 15 minutes
Servings: 4
Ingredients:
2 eggs
1 cup malty beer
1 cup all-purpose flour
½ cup cornstarch
1 teaspoon garlic powder
Salt and pepper, to taste
4 (4-ounce / 113-g) cod fillets
Cooking spray
Directions:
Mix the eggs with the beer in a shallow bowl. In another shallow bowl, thoroughly combine the flour and cornstarch. Sprinkle with the garlic powder, salt, and pepper.
Dredge each cod fillet in the flour mixture, then in the egg mixture. Dip each piece of fish in the flour mixture a second time.
Spritz the air fry basket with cooking spray. Arrange the cod fillets in the basket in a single layer.
Select Air Fry, Convection, set temperature to 400ºF (205ºC), and set time to 15 minutes.
Flip the fillets halfway through the cooking time. Let the fish cool for 5 minutes and serve.
Nutrition:
Calories: 189
Carbs: 11g
Fat: 14g
Protein: 15g

270. Tuna Lettuce Wraps

Preparation time: 10 minutes
Cooking time: 7 minutes

Servings: 4
Ingredients:
1 pound (454 g) fresh tuna steak, cut into 1-inch cubes
2 garlic cloves, minced
1 tablespoon grated fresh ginger
½ teaspoon toasted sesame oil
4 low-sodium whole-wheat tortillas
2 cups shredded romaine lettuce
1 red bell pepper, thinly sliced
¼ cup low-fat mayonnaise
Directions:
Combine the tuna cubes, garlic, ginger, and sesame oil in a medium bowl and toss until well coated. Allow sitting for 10 minutes.
When ready, place the tuna cubes in the air fry basket.
Select Air Fry, Convection, set temperature to 390ºF (199ºC), and set time to 6 minutes.
After that, remove the tuna cubes from the oven to a plate.
Put the tortillas on a flat working surface, top each tortilla evenly with the cooked tuna, lettuce, bell pepper, and finish with the mayonnaise to make the wraps. Roll them up and serve immediately.
Nutrition:
Calories: 300
Carbs: 0g
Fat: 0g
Protein: 0g

271. Tilapia Meunière with Vegetables

Preparation time: 10 minutes
Cooking time: 20 minutes
Servings: 4
Ingredients:
10 ounces (283 g) Yukon Gold potatoes, sliced ¼-inch thick
5 tablespoons unsalted butter, melted, divided
1 teaspoon kosher salt, divided
4 (8-ounce / 227-g) tilapia fillets
½ pound (227 g) green beans, trimmed
Juice of 1 lemon
2 tablespoons chopped fresh parsley, for garnish
Directions:
Drizzle the potatoes with 2 tablespoons of melted butter and ¼ teaspoon of kosher salt in a large bowl. Transfer the potatoes to the sheet pan.
Select Roast, Convection, set temperature to 375ºF (190ºC), and set time to 20 minutes.
Meanwhile, season both sides of the fillets with ½ teaspoon of kosher salt. Put the green beans in the medium bowl and sprinkle with the remaining ¼ teaspoon of kosher salt and 1 tablespoon of butter, tossing to coat.
After 10 minutes, remove the pan and push the potatoes to one side. Put the fillets in the middle of the pan and add the green beans on the other side. Drizzle the rest of the 2 tablespoons of butter over the fillets. Return it and cook until the fish flakes easily with a fork, and the green beans are crisp-tender.
Once cooked, remove and drizzle the lemon juice over the fillets and sprinkle the parsley on top for garnish. Serve hot.
Nutrition:
Calories: 172
Carbs: 24g
Fat: 2g
Protein: 24g

272. Glazed Tuna and Fruit Kebabs

Preparation time: 15 minutes
Cooking time: 10 minutes
Servings: 4
Ingredients:
Kebabs:
1-pound (454 g) tuna steaks, cut into 1-inch cubes
½ cup canned pineapple chunks, drained, juice reserved
½ cup large red grapes
Marinade:
1 tablespoon honey
1 teaspoon olive oil
2 teaspoons grated fresh ginger
Pinch cayenne pepper
Special Equipment:
4 metal skewers
Directions:
Make the kebabs: Thread, alternating tuna cubes, pineapple chunks, and red grapes, onto the metal skewers.
Make the marinade: Whisk the honey, olive oil, ginger, and cayenne pepper in a small bowl. Brush the marinade generously over the kebabs and allow to sit for 10 minutes.
When ready, transfer the kebabs to the air fry basket.
Select Air Fry, Convection, set temperature to 370ºF (188ºC), and set time to 10 minutes.
After 5 minutes, remove and flip the kebabs and brush with the remaining marinade. Return the basket to the oven and continue cooking for an additional 5 minutes.
Remove, and discard any remaining marinade. Serve hot.
Nutrition:
Calories: 319
Carbs: 0g
Fat: 0g
Protein: 0g

273. Snapper with Tomatoes and Olives

Preparation time: 9 minutes
Cooking time: 18 minutes
Servings: 4
Ingredients:
2 tablespoons extra-virgin olive oil
2 large garlic cloves, minced
½ onion, finely chopped
1 (14.5-ounce / 411-g) can diced tomatoes, drained
¼ cup sliced green olives
3 tablespoons capers, divided
2 tablespoons chopped fresh parsley, divided
½ teaspoon dried oregano
4 (6-ounce / 170-g) snapper fillets
½ teaspoon kosher salt

Directions:

Grease the sheet pan generously with olive oil, then place the pan on the roast position.

Select Roast, Convection, set temperature to 375ºF (190ºC), and set time to 18 minutes.

Remove the pan and add the garlic and onion to the pan's olive oil, stirring to coat, then return it to the air fryer oven. Set within 2 minutes.

Remove, then stir in the tomatoes, olives, 1½ tablespoons of capers, 1 tablespoon of parsley, and oregano. Return it and cook within 6 minutes until heated through.

Meanwhile, rub the fillets with the salt on both sides.

After another 6 minutes, remove and put the fillets in the center of the sheet pan, and spoon the sauce.

Return it and continue cooking, or until the fish is flaky.

When cooked, remove and scatter the remaining 1½ tablespoons of capers and 1 tablespoon of parsley on top of the fillets, then serve.

Nutrition:

Calories: 328
Carbs: 4g
Fat: 16g
Protein: 36g

274. Air Fried Cod Fillets

Preparation time: 15 minutes
Cooking time: 12 minutes
Servings: 4

Ingredients:

4 cod fillets
¼ teaspoon fine sea salt
1 teaspoon cayenne pepper
¼ teaspoon ground black pepper
½ cup fresh Italian parsley, coarsely chopped
½ cup non-dairy milk
4 garlic cloves, minced
1 Italian pepper, chopped
1 teaspoon dried basil
½ teaspoon dried oregano
Cooking spray

Directions:

Lightly grease a baking dish using cooking spray.

Season the fillets with salt, cayenne pepper, and black pepper.

Pulse the remaining ingredients in a food processor, then transfer the mixture to a shallow bowl. Coat the fillets with the mixture.

Select Air Fry, Convection, set temperature to 375ºF (190ºC), and set time to 12 minutes.

Remove once it's done and serve on a plate.

Nutrition:

Calories: 80
Carbs: 0g
Fat: 3g
Protein: 14g

275. Sticky Hoisin Tuna

Preparation time: 15 minutes
Cooking time: 5 minutes
Servings: 4

Ingredients:

½ cup hoisin sauce
2 tablespoons of rice wine vinegar
2 teaspoons sesame oil
2 teaspoons dried lemongrass
1 teaspoon garlic powder
¼ teaspoon red pepper flakes
½ small onion quartered and thinly sliced
8 ounces (227 g) fresh tuna, cut into 1-inch cubes
Cooking spray
3 cups cooked jasmine rice

Directions:

Whisk the hoisin sauce, vinegar, sesame oil, lemongrass, garlic powder, and red pepper flakes in a small bowl.

Add the sliced onion and tuna cubes and gently toss until the fish is evenly coated.

Arrange the coated tuna cubes in the air fry basket in a single layer.

Select Air Fry, Convection, set temperature to 390ºF (199ºC), and set time to 5 minutes.

Flip the fish halfway through the cooking time.

Continue cooking for 1 minute, if necessary. Remove, then serve over hot jasmine rice.

Nutrition:

Calories: 273
Carbs: 9g
Fat: 9g
Protein: 0g

276. Parmesan-Crusted Halibut Fillets

Preparation time: 5 minutes
Cooking time: 10 minutes
Servings: 4

Ingredients:

2 medium-sized halibut fillets
Dash of tabasco sauce
1 teaspoon curry powder
½ teaspoon ground coriander
½ teaspoon hot paprika
Kosher salt and freshly cracked mixed peppercorns, to taste
2 eggs
1½ tablespoons olive oil
½ cup grated Parmesan cheese

Directions:

On a clean work surface, drizzle the halibut fillets with the tabasco sauce. Sprinkle with the curry powder, coriander, hot paprika, salt, and cracked mixed peppercorns. Set aside.

Beat the eggs until frothy in a shallow bowl. In another shallow bowl, combine the olive oil and Parmesan cheese.

One at a time, dredge the halibut fillets in the beaten eggs, shaking off any excess, then roll them over the Parmesan cheese until evenly coated.

Arrange the halibut fillets in the air fry basket in a single layer.

Select Roast, Convection, set temperature to 365ºF (185ºC), and set time to 10 minutes.

Cool for 5 minutes before serving.

Nutrition:

Calories: 308
Carbs: 6g
Fat: 14g
Protein: 38g

277. Crispy Fish Sticks

Preparation time: 10 minutes
Cooking time: 6 minutes
Servings: 8

Ingredients:

8 ounces (227 g) fish fillets (pollock or cod), cut into ½ × 3 inches strips
Salt, to taste (optional)
½ cup plain bread crumbs
Cooking spray

Directions:

Season the fish strips with salt to taste, if desired.
Put the bread crumbs on a plate, then roll the fish in the bread crumbs until well coated. Spray all sides of the fish with cooking spray. Transfer to the air fry basket in a single layer.
Select Air Fry, Convection, set temperature to 400ºF (205ºC), and set time to 6 minutes.
When cooked, the fish sticks should be golden brown and crispy. Serve hot.

Nutrition:

Calories: 220
Carbs: 20g
Fat: 10g
Protein: 11g

278. Herbed Salmon with Roasted Asparagus

Preparation time: 5 minutes
Cooking time: 12 minutes
Servings: 2

Ingredients:

2 teaspoons olive oil
2 (5-ounce / 142-g) salmon fillets, with skin
Salt
ground black pepper
1 bunch asparagus, trimmed
1 teaspoon dried tarragon
1 teaspoon dried chives
Fresh lemon wedges, for serving

Directions:

Massage the olive oil all over the salmon fillets.
Sprinkle with salt and pepper to taste.
Put the asparagus on a foil-lined baking sheet and place the salmon fillets on top, skin-side down.
Select Roast, Convection, set temperature to 425ºF (220ºC), and set time to 12 minutes.
When cooked, the fillets should register 145ºF (63ºC) on an instant-read thermometer.
Remove and cut the salmon fillets in half crosswise, then use a metal spatula to lift flesh from the skin and transfer to a serving plate.
Discard the skin and drizzle the salmon fillets with additional olive oil. Scatter with the herbs.
Serve the salmon fillets with roasted asparagus spears and lemon wedges on the side.

Nutrition:

Calories: 72
Carbs: 8g
Fat: 3g
Protein: 6g

279. Easy Salmon Patties

Preparation time: 5 minutes
Cooking time: 11 minutes
Servings: 6

Ingredients:

1 (14.75-ounce / 418-g) can Alaskan pink salmon, drained and bones removed
½ cup bread crumbs
1 egg, whisked
2 scallions, diced
1 teaspoon garlic powder
Salt and pepper, to taste
Cooking spray

Directions:

Stir the salmon, bread crumbs, whisked egg, scallions, garlic powder, salt, and pepper in a large bowl until well incorporated.
Split the salmon mixture into six portions and form each into a patty with your hands.
Arrange the salmon patties in the air fry basket and spritz them with cooking spray.
Select Air Fry, Convection, set temperature to 400ºF (205ºC), and set time to 10 minutes.
Flip the patties once halfway through.
Remove the oven and serve on a plate.

Nutrition:

Calories: 196
Carbs: 15g
Fat: 9g
Protein: 16g

280. Breaded Fish Fillets

Preparation time: 20 minutes
Cooking time: 7 minutes
Servings: 4

Ingredients:

1-pound (454 g) fish fillets
1 tablespoon course brown mustard
1 teaspoon Worcestershire sauce
½ teaspoon hot sauce
Salt, to taste
Cooking spray
Crumb Coating:
¾ cup panko bread crumbs
¼ cup stone-ground cornmeal
¼ teaspoon salt

Directions:

On your cutting board, cut the fish fillets crosswise into slices, about 1 inch wide.
In a small bowl, stir the mustard, Worcestershire sauce, and hot sauce to make a paste and rub this paste on all the fillets' sides. Season with salt to taste.
In a shallow bowl, thoroughly combine all the crumb coating ingredients and spread them on a sheet of wax paper.
Roll the fish fillets in the crumb mixture until thickly coated. Spritz all sides of the fish with cooking spray, then arrange them in the air fry basket in a single layer.
Select Air Fry, Convection, set temperature to 400ºF (205ºC), and set time to 7 minutes.
Remove and serve warm.

Nutrition:

Calories: 177
Carbs: 0g

Fat: 0g
Protein: 0g

281. Basil Salmon with Tomatoes

Preparation time: 10 minutes
Cooking time: 15 minutes
Servings: 4

Ingredients:

4 (6-ounce / 170-g) salmon fillets, patted dry
1 teaspoon kosher salt, divided
2 pints cherry, divided
3 tablespoons extra-virgin olive oil, divided
2 garlic cloves, minced
1 small red bell pepper, chopped
2 tablespoons chopped fresh basil, divided

Directions:

Season both sides of the salmon with ½ teaspoon of kosher salt.
Put about half of the tomatoes in a large bowl, along with the remaining ½ teaspoon of kosher salt, 2 tablespoons of olive oil, garlic, bell pepper, and 1 tablespoon basil. Toss to coat and then transfer to the sheet pan.
Set the salmon fillets on the sheet pan, skin-side down. Brush them with the remaining 1 tablespoon of olive oil.
Select Roast, Convection, set temperature to 375ºF (190ºC), and set time to 15 minutes.
After 7 minutes, remove the pan and fold in the remaining tomatoes. Return to the oven and cook again.
When cooked, remove and serve sprinkled with the remaining 1 tablespoon of basil.

Nutrition:

Calories: 248
Carbs: 3g
Fat: 10g
Protein: 35g

282. Chili Prawns

Preparation time: 10 minutes
Cooking time: 8 minutes
Servings: 2

Ingredients:

8 prawns, cleaned
Salt and black pepper, to taste
½ teaspoon ground cayenne pepper
½ teaspoon garlic powder
½ teaspoon ground cumin
½ teaspoon red chili flakes
Cooking spray

Directions:

Spritz an air fryer basket with cooking spray.
Toss the remaining ingredients in a large bowl until the prawns are well coated.
Spread the coated prawns evenly in the air fryer basket and spray them with cooking spray.
Cook at 340ºF (171ºC) for 8 minutes. Flip the prawns halfway through the cooking time.
When done, the prawns should be pink. Remove the prawns from the air fryer oven to a plate.

Nutrition:

Calories: 90
Carbs: 0g
Fat: 3g
Protein: 14g

283. Tex-Mex Salmon Bowl

Preparation time: 15 minutes
Cooking time: 12 minutes
Servings: 4

Ingredients:

12 ounces (340 g) salmon fillets, cut into 1½-inch cubes
1 red onion, chopped
1 jalapeño pepper, minced
1 red bell pepper, chopped
¼ cup low-sodium salsa
2 teaspoons peanut oil or safflower oil
2 tablespoons low-sodium tomato juice
1 teaspoon chili powder

Directions:

Mix the salmon cubes, red onion, jalapeño, red bell pepper, salsa, peanut oil, tomato juice, chili powder in a medium metal bowl, and stir until well incorporated.
Place the metal bowl into the air fryer oven—Cook at 370ºF (188ºC) for 12 minutes.
Stir the ingredients once halfway through the cooking time.
The salmon should be cooked through, and the veggies should be fork-tender. Serve warm.

Nutrition:

Calories: 265
Carbs: 27g
Fat: 4g
Protein: 31g

284. Shrimp and Cherry Tomato Kebabs

Preparation time: 15 minutes
Cooking time: 5 minutes
Servings: 4

Ingredients:

1½ pounds (680 g) jumbo shrimp, cleaned, shelled, and deveined
1-pound (454 g) cherry tomatoes
2 tablespoons butter, melted
1 tablespoons Sriracha sauce
Sea salt
ground black pepper
1 teaspoon dried parsley flakes
½ teaspoon dried basil
½ teaspoon dried oregano
½ teaspoon mustard seeds
½ teaspoon marjoram
Special Equipment:
4 to 6 wooden skewers, soaked

Directions:

Put all the fixings in a large bowl and toss to coat well.
Make the kebabs: Thread, alternating jumbo shrimp and cherry tomatoes, onto the wooden skewers.
Place the kebabs in an air fryer basket.
Cook at 400ºF (205ºC) for 5 minutes.
Let the shrimp and cherry tomato kebabs cool for 5 minutes and serves hot.

Nutrition:

Calories: 124
Carbs: 2g

Fat: 1g
Protein: 23g

285. Breaded Scallops

Preparation time: 5 minutes
Cooking time: 7 minutes
Servings: 4

Ingredients:

1 egg
3 tablespoons flour
1 cup bread crumbs
1 pound (454 g) fresh scallops
2 tablespoons olive oil
Salt and black pepper, to taste

Directions:

In a bowl, lightly beat the egg. Place the flour and bread crumbs into separate shallow dishes.
Dredge the scallops in the flour and shake off any excess. Dip the flour-coated scallops in the beaten egg and roll in the bread crumbs.
Brush the scallops generously with olive oil and season with salt and pepper, to taste. Transfer the scallops to an air fryer basket.
Cook at 360ºF (182ºC) for 7 minutes.
Flip the scallops halfway through the cooking time.
Let the scallops cool for 5 minutes and serve.

Nutrition:

Calories: 180
Carbs: 18g
Fat: 8g
Protein: 9g

286. Baked Tilapia with Garlic Aioli

Preparation time: 5 minutes
Cooking time: 15 minutes
Servings: 4

Ingredients:

Tilapia:
4 tilapia fillets
1 tablespoon extra-virgin olive oil
1 teaspoon garlic powder
1 teaspoon paprika
1 teaspoon dried basil
A pinch of lemon-pepper seasoning
Garlic Aioli:
2 garlic cloves, minced
1 tablespoon mayonnaise
Juice of ½ lemon
1 teaspoon extra-virgin olive oil
Salt and pepper, to taste

Directions:

Brush each side of the fillet with the olive oil on a clean work surface. Sprinkle with the garlic powder, paprika, basil, and lemon-pepper seasoning. Place the fillets in an air fryer basket.
Cook at 400ºF (205ºC) for 15 minutes.
Flip the fillets halfway through.
Meanwhile, make the garlic aioli: Whisk the garlic, mayo, lemon juice, olive oil, salt, and pepper in a small bowl until smooth.
Remove the fish from the air fryer oven and serve with the garlic aioli on the side.

Nutrition:

Calories: 150
Carbs: 1g
Fat: 7g
Protein: 21g

287. Caesar Shrimp Salad

Preparation time: 15 minutes
Cooking time: 15 minutes
Servings: 4

Ingredients:

½ baguette, cut into 1-inch cubes (about 2½ cups)
4 tablespoons extra-virgin olive oil, divided
¼ teaspoon granulated garlic
¼ teaspoon kosher salt
¾ cup Caesar dressing, divided
2 romaine lettuce hearts, cut in half lengthwise and ends trimmed
1 pound (454 g) medium shrimp, peeled and deveined
2 ounces (57 g) Parmesan cheese, coarsely grated

Directions:

Put the bread cubes in a bowl to make the croutons and drizzle 3 tablespoons of olive oil over the top. Season with granulated garlic and salt and toss to coat. Transfer to an air fryer basket.
Cook at 400ºF (205ºC) for 4 minutes.
Toss the croutons halfway through the cooking time. When done, remove the air fryer basket from the air fryer oven and set aside.
Brush 2 tablespoons of Caesar dressing on the cut side of the lettuce. Set aside.
Toss the shrimp with the ¼ cup of Caesar dressing in a large bowl until well coated. Set aside.
Coat a sheet pan with the remaining 1 tablespoon of olive oil. Arrange the romaine halves on the coated pan, cut side down. Brush the tops with the remaining 2 tablespoons of Caesar dressing.
Cook at 375ºF (190ºC) for 10 minutes in the air fryer oven.
After 5 minutes, remove and flip the romaine halves. Spoon the shrimp around the lettuce. Continue cooking.
Remove the sheet pan from the air fryer oven. If they are not entirely cooked through, roast for another 1 minute.
On each of four plates, put a romaine half. Divide the shrimp among the plates and top with croutons and grated Parmesan cheese. Serve immediately.

Nutrition:

Calories: 290
Carbs: 15g
Fat: 12g
Protein: 36g

288. Baked Flounder Fillets

Preparation time: 8 minutes
Cooking time: 12 minutes
Servings: 2

Ingredients:

2 flounder fillets, patted dry
1 egg
½ teaspoon Worcestershire sauce
¼ cup almond flour
¼ cup coconut flour
½ teaspoon coarse sea salt

½ teaspoon lemon pepper
¼ teaspoon chili powder
Cooking spray
Directions:
Whisk the egg with Worcestershire sauce until well incorporated in a shallow bowl.
In another bowl, thoroughly combine the almond flour, coconut flour, sea salt, lemon pepper, and chili powder.
Dredge the fillets in the egg mixture, shaking off any excess, then roll in the flour mixture to coat well.
Spritz an air fryer basket with cooking spray. Place the fillets in the basket.
Cook at 390ºF (199ºC) for 12 minutes.
After 7 minutes, remove and flip the fillets and spray with cooking spray. Continue to again for 5 minutes, or until the fish is flaky.
Serve warm.
Nutrition:
Calories: 213
Carbs: 2g
Fat: 10g
Protein: 27g

289. Crispy Crab and Fish Cakes

Preparation time: 15 minutes
Cooking time: 12 minutes
Servings: 4
Ingredients:
8 ounces (227 g) imitation crab meat
4 ounces (113 g) leftover cooked fish (such as cod, pollock, or haddock)
2 tablespoons minced celery
2 tablespoons minced green onion
2 tablespoons light mayonnaise
1 tablespoon plus 2 teaspoons Worcestershire sauce
¾ cup crushed saltine cracker crumbs
2 teaspoons dried parsley flakes
1 teaspoon prepared yellow mustard
½ teaspoon garlic powder
½ teaspoon dried dill weed, crushed
½ teaspoon Old Bay seasoning
½ cup panko bread crumbs
Cooking spray
Directions:
Pulse the crab meat and fish in a food processor until finely chopped.
Transfer the meat mixture to a large bowl, along with the celery, green onion, mayo, Worcestershire sauce, cracker crumbs, parsley flakes, mustard, garlic powder, dill weed, and Old Bay seasoning. Stir to mix well.
Scoop out the meat mixture and form into 8 equal-sized patties with your hands.
Put the panko bread crumbs on a dish plate. Roll the patties in the bread crumbs until they are evenly coated on both sides. Put the patties in an air fryer basket and spritz them with cooking spray.
Cook at 390ºF (199ºC) for 12 minutes.
Flip the patties halfway through the cooking time.
Divide the patties among four plates and serve.
Nutrition:
Calories: 218
Carbs: 13g
Fat: 4g
Protein: 16g

290. Breaded Calamari with Lemon

Preparation time: 5 minutes
Cooking time: 12 minutes
Servings: 4
Ingredients:
2 large eggs
2 garlic cloves, minced
½ cup cornstarch
1 cup bread crumbs
1-pound (454 g) calamari rings
Cooking spray
1 lemon, sliced
Directions:
Whisk the eggs with minced garlic in a small bowl.
Place the cornstarch and bread crumbs into separate shallow dishes.
Dredge the calamari rings in the cornstarch, then dip in the egg mixture, shaking off any excess, finally roll them in the bread crumbs to coat well. Let the calamari rings sit for 10 minutes in the refrigerator.
Spritz an air fryer basket with cooking spray.
Transfer the calamari rings to the pan.
Cook at 390ºF (199ºC) for 12 minutes.
Stir the calamari rings once halfway through the cooking time.
Serve the calamari rings with the lemon slices sprinkled on top.
Nutrition:
Calories: 98
Carbs: 0g
Fat: 1g
Protein: 21g

291. Browned Shrimp Patties

Preparation time: 15 minutes
Cooking time: 12 minutes
Servings: 4
Ingredients:
½ pound (227 g) raw shrimp, shelled, deveined, and chopped finely
2 cups cooked sushi rice
¼ cup chopped red bell pepper
¼ cup chopped celery
¼ cup chopped green onion
2 teaspoons Worcestershire sauce
½ teaspoon salt
½ teaspoon garlic powder
½ teaspoon Old Bay seasoning
½ cup plain bread crumbs
Cooking spray
Directions:
Put all the fixings except the bread crumbs and oil in a large bowl and stir to incorporate.
Scoop out the shrimp mixture and shape into 8 equal-sized patties with your hands, no more than ½-inch thick. Roll out the patties in the bread crumbs on a plate and spray both sides with cooking spray.
Place the patties in an air fryer basket.
Cook at 390ºF (199ºC) for 12 minutes.
Turn over the patties halfway through the cooking time.

The outside should be crispy brown. Divide the patties among four plates and serve warm.

Nutrition:

Calories: 130
Carbs: 14g
Fat: 5g
Protein: 9g

292. Cajun and Lemon Pepper Cod

Preparation time: 5 minutes
Cooking time: 12 minutes
Servings: 2

Ingredients:

1 tablespoon Cajun seasoning
1 teaspoon salt
½ teaspoon lemon pepper
½ teaspoon freshly ground black pepper
2 (8-ounce / 227-g) cod fillets, cut to fit into an air fryer basket
Cooking spray
2 tablespoons unsalted butter, melted
1 lemon, cut into 4 wedges

Directions:

Spritz an air fryer basket with cooking spray.
Thoroughly combine the Cajun seasoning, salt, lemon pepper, and black pepper in a small bowl. Rub this mixture all over the cod fillets until coated.
Put the fillets in an air fryer basket and brush the melted butter over both sides of each fillet.
Cook at 360ºF (182ºC) for 12 minutes.
Turn over the fillets halfway through the cooking time.
Remove the fillets from the air fryer oven and serve with fresh lemon wedges.

Nutrition:

Calories: 140
Carbs: 2g
Fat: 4g
Protein: 25g

293. Garlic Butter Shrimp Scampi

Preparation time: 5 minutes
Cooking time: 8 minutes
Servings: 4

Ingredients:

Sauce:
¼ cup unsalted butter
2 tablespoons fish stock or chicken broth
2 cloves garlic, minced
2 tablespoons chopped fresh basil leaves
1 tablespoon lemon juice
1 tablespoon fresh parsley, chopped
1 teaspoon red pepper flakes
Shrimp:
1 pound (454 g) large shrimp, peeled and deveined, tails removed
Fresh basil sprigs, for garnish

Directions:

Put all the fixings for the sauce in a baking pan and stir to incorporate.
Cook at 350ºF (180ºC) for 8 minutes in the air fryer oven.
After 3 minutes, remove and add the shrimp to the baking pan, flipping to coat in the sauce, then cook again for 5 minutes until the shrimp are pink and opaque. Stir the shrimp twice during cooking.
Serve garnished with the parsley and basil sprigs.

Nutrition:

Calories: 85
Carbs: 1g
Fat: 8g
Protein: 23g

294. Butter-Wine Baked Salmon

Preparation time: 5 minutes
Cooking time: 10 minutes
Servings: 4

Ingredients:

4 tablespoons butter, melted
2 cloves garlic, minced
Sea salt
ground black pepper
¼ cup dry white wine
1 tablespoon lime juice
1 teaspoon smoked paprika
½ teaspoon onion powder
4 salmon steaks
Cooking spray

Directions:

Put all the fixings except the salmon and oil in a shallow dish and stir to mix well.
Add the salmon steaks, turning to coat well on both sides. Transfer the salmon to the refrigerator to marinate for 30 minutes.
When ready, put the salmon steaks in an air fryer basket, discarding any excess marinade. Spray the salmon steaks with cooking spray.
Cook at 360ºF (182ºC) for 10 minutes.
Flip the salmon steaks halfway through. When done, serve warm.

Nutrition:

Calories: 250
Carbs: 2g
Fat: 16g
Protein: 24g

295. Crab Ratatouille with Eggplant and Tomatoes

Preparation time: 15 minutes
Cooking time: 13 minutes
Servings: 4

Ingredients:

1½ cups peeled and cubed eggplant
2 large tomatoes, chopped
1 red bell pepper, chopped
1 onion, chopped
1 tablespoon olive oil
½ teaspoon dried basil
½ teaspoon dried thyme
Pinch salt
Freshly ground black pepper, to taste
1½ cups cooked crab meat

Directions:

In a metal bowl, stir the eggplant, tomatoes, bell pepper, onion, olive oil, basil, and thyme. Season with salt and pepper.
Place the metal bowl into the air fryer oven—Cook at 400ºF (205ºC) for 13 minutes.

After 9 minutes, remove the bowl from the air fryer oven.
Add the crabmeat, stir well, and continue roasting for another 4 minutes, or until the vegetables are softened, and the ratatouille is bubbling. Serve warm.

Nutrition:

Calories: 109
Carbs: 14g
Fat: 5g
Protein: 2g

296. Piri-Piri King Prawns

Preparation time: 10 minutes
Cooking time: 8 minutes
Servings: 2

Ingredients:

12 king prawns, rinsed
1 tablespoon coconut oil
Salt and ground black pepper, to taste
1 teaspoon onion powder
1 teaspoon garlic paste
1 teaspoon curry powder
½ teaspoon Piri-Piri powder
½ teaspoon cumin powder

Directions:

Mix all the fixings in a large bowl and toss until the prawns are completely coated. Place the prawns in an air fryer basket.
Cook at 360ºF (182ºC) for 8 minutes.
Flip the prawns halfway through the cooking time.
Serve hot.

Nutrition:

Calories: 147
Carbs: 10g
Fat: 7g
Protein: 11g

297. Bacon-Wrapped Shrimp

Preparation time: 5 minutes
Cooking time: 5 minutes
Servings: 4

Ingredients:

1¼ pound tiger shrimp, peeled and deveined
1-pound bacon

Directions:

Wrap all shrimp individually with a slice of bacon.
Refrigerate for about 20 minutes.
Preheat the air fryer oven to 390 degrees F.
Arrange the shrimp in the oven rack. Put the rack on the middle shelf —Cook for about 5-7 minutes.

Nutrition:

Calories: 40
Carbs: 1g
Fat: 40g
Protein: 30g

298. Air Fryer Salmon

Preparation time: 15 minutes
Cooking time: 10 minutes
Servings: 2

Ingredients:

½ tsp salt
½ tsp garlic powder
½ tsp smoked paprika
Salmon

Directions:

Mix spices and sprinkle onto salmon. Place seasoned salmon into the air fryer oven.
Set temperature to 400°F, and set time to 10 minutes.
Serve.

Nutrition:

Calories: 259
Carbs: 0g
Fat: 12g
Protein: 33g

299. Sweet and Savory Breaded Shrimp

Preparation time: 5 minutes
Cooking time: 20 minutes
Servings: 2

Ingredients:

½ pound of fresh shrimp, peeled from their shells and rinsed
2 raw eggs
½ cup of breadcrumbs
½ white onion, peeled and rinsed and finely chopped
1 teaspoon of ginger-garlic paste
½ teaspoon of turmeric powder
½ teaspoon of red chili powder
½ teaspoon of cumin powder
½ teaspoon of black pepper powder
½ teaspoon of dry mango powder
Pinch of salt

Directions:

Cover the air fryer oven basket with a tin foil, uncovered the edge to allow the air to circulate through the basket.
Preheat the air fryer oven to 350 degrees.
Whisk the eggs until fluffy in a large mixing bowl.
Dunk all the shrimp in the egg mixture, fully submerging.
Mix the bread crumbs with all the dry ingredients until evenly blended in a separate mixing bowl.
One by one, coat the egg-covered shrimp in the mixed dry ingredients fully covered, and place on the foil-lined air-fryer basket.
Set the air-fryer timer to 20 minutes.
Shake the handle of the air-fryer halfway through the cooking time so that the breaded shrimp jostles inside and fry-coverage is even.
After 20 minutes, when the fryer shuts off, the shrimp will be perfectly cooked, and their breaded crust golden-brown and delicious! Set on a serving dish to cool.

Nutrition:

Calories: 170
Carbs: 25g
Fat: 2g
Protein: 14g

300. Quick Paella

Preparation time: 7 minutes
Cooking time: 15 minutes
Servings: 4

Ingredients:

1 (10-ounce) package frozen cooked rice, thawed
1 (6-ounce) jar artichoke hearts, drained and chopped

¼ cup vegetable broth
½ teaspoon turmeric
½ teaspoon dried thyme
1 cup frozen cooked small shrimp
½ cup frozen baby peas
1 tomato, diced

Directions:

In a 6-by-6-by-2-inch pan, combine the rice, artichoke hearts, vegetable broth, turmeric, and thyme, and stir gently.
Place in the air fryer oven and bake for 8 to 9 minutes or until the rice is hot. Remove and gently stir in the shrimp, peas, and tomato.
Cook for 5 to 8 minutes or until the shrimp and peas are hot, and the paella is bubbling.

Nutrition:

Calories: 371
Carbs: 44g
Fat: 7g
Protein: 30g

301. Cilantro-Lime Fried Shrimp

Preparation time: 15 minutes
Cooking time: 10 minutes
Servings: 4

Ingredients:

1-pound raw shrimp, peeled and deveined with tails on or off
½ cup chopped fresh cilantro
Juice of 1 lime
1 egg
½ cup all-purpose flour
¾ cup bread crumbs
Salt
Pepper
Cooking oil
½ cup cocktail sauce (optional)

Directions:

Place the shrimp in a plastic bag and add the cilantro and lime juice. Seal the bag. Shake to combine. Marinate in the refrigerator for 30 minutes.
In a small bowl, beat the egg. In another small bowl, place the flour. Put all your bread crumbs in a bowl and season with salt and pepper to taste.
Spray the air fryer rack/basket with cooking oil.
Remove the shrimp from the plastic bag. Dip each in the flour, then the egg, and then the bread crumbs.
Place the shrimp in the air fryer oven. It is okay to stack them. Spray the shrimp with cooking oil—Cook for 4 minutes.
Flip the shrimp individually instead of shaking to keep the breading intact. Cook again within 4 minutes, or until crisp.
Cool before serving. Serve with cocktail sauce if desired.

Nutrition:

Calories: 112
Carbs: 2g
Fat: 5g
Protein: 17g

302. Lemony Tuna

Preparation time: 15 minutes
Cooking time: 10 minutes
Servings: 4

Ingredients:

2 (6-ounce) cans water-packed plain tuna
2 teaspoons Dijon mustard
½ cup breadcrumbs
1 tablespoon fresh lime juice
2 tablespoons fresh parsley, chopped
1 egg
Chefman of hot sauce
3 tablespoons canola oil
Salt
ground black pepper

Directions:

In a bowl, add the fish tuna, mustard, crumbs, citrus juice, parsley, and hot sauce and mix till well combined. Add a little canola oil if it seems too dry. Add egg, salt, and stir to combine. Make the patties from tuna mixture. Refrigerate the tuna patties for about 2 hours.
Preheat the air fryer oven to 355 degrees F. Cook for about 10-12 minutes.

Nutrition:

Calories: 297
Carbs: 0g
Fat: 2g
Protein: 27g

303. Grilled Soy Salmon Fillets

Preparation time: 5 minutes
Cooking time: 8 minutes
Servings: 4

Ingredients:

4 salmon fillets
1/4 teaspoon ground black pepper
1/2 teaspoon cayenne pepper
1/2 teaspoon salt
1 teaspoon onion powder
1 tablespoon fresh lemon juice
1/2 cup soy sauce
1/2 cup water
1 tablespoon honey
2 tablespoons extra-virgin olive oil

Directions:

Pat dry the salmon fillets using kitchen towels.
Season the salmon with black pepper, cayenne pepper, salt, and onion powder.
To make the marinade, combine the lemon juice, soy sauce, water, honey, and olive oil. Marinate the salmon for at least 2 hours in your refrigerator.
Arrange the fish fillets on a grill basket in your air fryer oven.
Bake at 330 degrees for 8 to 9 minutes, or until salmon fillets is easily flaked with a fork.
Work with batches and serve warm.

Nutrition:

Calories: 241
Carbs: 0g
Fat: 14g
Protein: 28g

304. Scallops and Spring Veggies

Preparation time: 15 minutes
Cooking time: 8 minutes
Servings: 4

Ingredients:
½ pound asparagus ends trimmed, cut into 2-inch pieces
1 cup sugar snap peas
1-pound sea scallops
1 tablespoon lemon juice
2 teaspoons olive oil
½ teaspoon dried thyme
Pinch salt
ground black pepper
Directions:
Put the asparagus plus sugar snap peas in your air fryer oven basket.
Cook within 2 to 3 minutes or until the vegetables are just starting to get tender.
Meanwhile, check the scallops for a small muscle attached to the side, and pull it off and discard it.
Toss the scallops with lemon juice, olive oil, thyme, salt, and pepper in a medium bowl and then place it into the oven rack on top of the vegetables.
Steam for 5 to 7 minutes. Until the scallops are just firm, and the vegetables are tender. Serve immediately.
Nutrition:
Calories: 293
Carbs: 28g
Fat: 15g
Protein: 10g

305. Fried Calamari

Preparation time: 8 minutes
Cooking time: 7 minutes
Servings: 8
Ingredients:
½ tsp. salt
½ tsp. Old Bay seasoning
1/3 C. plain cornmeal
½ C. semolina flour
½ C. almond flour
5-6 C. olive oil
1 ½ pounds baby squid
Directions:
Rinse squid in cold water and slice tentacles, keeping just ¼-inch of the hood in one piece.
Combine 1-2 pinches of pepper, salt, Old Bay seasoning, cornmeal, and both flours. Dredge squid pieces into the flour mixture and place them into the air fryer oven.
Spray liberally with olive oil. Cook 15 minutes at 345 degrees till coating turns a golden brown.
Nutrition:
Calories: 158
Carbs: 2g
Fat: 1g
Protein: 32g

306. Soy and Ginger Shrimp

Preparation time: 8 minutes
Cooking time: 10 minutes
Servings: 4
Ingredients:
2 tablespoons olive oil
2 tablespoons scallions, finely chopped
2 cloves garlic, chopped
1 teaspoon fresh ginger, grated
1 tablespoon dry white wine
1 tablespoon balsamic vinegar
1/4 cup soy sauce
1 tablespoon sugar
1-pound shrimp
Salt and ground black pepper, to taste
Directions:
To make the marinade, warm the oil in a saucepan; cook all ingredients, except the shrimp, salt, and black pepper. Now, let it cool.
Marinate the shrimp, covered, at least an hour, in the refrigerator.
After that, bake the shrimp at 350 degrees F for 8 to 10 minutes (depending on the size), turning once or twice. Season prepared shrimp with salt and black pepper and serve right away.
Nutrition:
Calories: 119
Carbs: 2g
Fat: 1g
Protein: 24g

307. Crispy Cheesy Fish Fingers

Preparation time: 15 minutes
Cooking time: 20 minutes
Servings: 4
Ingredients:
Large codfish filet, cut into 1 ½-inch strip
2 raw eggs
½ cup of breadcrumbs
2 tablespoons of shredded or powdered parmesan cheese
1 tablespoon of shredded cheddar cheese
Pinch of salt and pepper
Directions:
Cover the air fryer oven basket with a foil, leave the edges uncovered to circulate the air through the basket.
Preheat the air fryer oven to 350 degrees.
Whisk the eggs until fluffy in a large mixing bowl.
Dunk all the fish strips in the beaten eggs, fully submerging.
Mix the bread crumbs with the parmesan, cheddar, salt, and pepper until evenly mixed in a separate mixing bowl.
One by one, coat the egg-covered fish strips in the mixed dry ingredients so that they're fully covered, and place on the foil-lined oven rack. Place the in on the middle-shelf.
Set the air-fryer timer to 20 minutes. Halfway through the cooking time, shake the handle of the air-fryer.
Remove and set on a serving dish to cool.
Nutrition:
Calories: 215
Carbs: 17g
Fat: 12g
Protein: 0g

308. Panko-Crusted Tilapia

Preparation time: 5 minutes
Cooking time: 10 minutes
Servings: 3

Ingredients:

2 tsp. Italian seasoning
2 tsp. lemon pepper
1/3 C. panko breadcrumbs
1/3 C. egg whites
1/3 C. almond flour
3 tilapia fillets
Olive oil

Directions:

Place panko, egg whites, and flour into separate bowls. Mix lemon pepper and Italian seasoning in with breadcrumbs.

Pat tilapia fillets dry. Dredge in flour, egg, then breadcrumb mixture.

Add to the Oven rack and spray lightly with olive oil.

Cook 10-11 minutes at 400 degrees, making sure to flip halfway through cooking. Serve.

Nutrition:

Calories: 180
Carbs: 15g
Fat: 8g
Protein: 11g

309. Fish Cakes with Mango Relish

Preparation time: 5 minutes
Cooking time: 10 minutes
Servings: 4

Ingredients:

1 lb. White Fish Fillets
3 tbsps. Ground Coconut
1 Ripened Mango
½ tsp. Chili Paste
Fresh Parsley
1 Green Onion
1 Lime
1 Tsp Salt
1 Egg

Directions:

To make the relish, peel and dice the mango into cubes. Combine with a half teaspoon of chili paste, a tablespoon of parsley, and the zest and juice of half a lime.

In a food processor, pulse the fish until it forms a smooth texture. Place into a bowl and add the salt, egg, chopped green onion, parsley, two tablespoons of the coconut, and the remainder of the chili paste and lime zest and juice. Combine well

Portion the mixture into 10 equal balls and flatten them into small patties. Pour the reserved tablespoon of the coconut onto a dish and roll the patties over to coat.

Preheat the Air fryer oven to 390 degrees

Place the fish cakes into the air fryer oven and cook for 8 minutes.

Serve hot with mango relish

Nutrition:

Calories: 30
Carbs: 5g
Fat: 0g
Protein: 0g

310. Sesame Seeds Coated Fish

Preparation time: 15 minutes
Cooking time: 8 minutes
Servings: 5

Ingredients:

3 tablespoons plain flour
2 eggs
½ cup sesame seeds, toasted
½ cup breadcrumbs
1/8 teaspoon dried rosemary, crushed
Pinch of salt
Pinch of black pepper
3 tablespoons olive oil
5 frozen fish fillets (white fish of your choice)

Directions:

In a shallow dish, place flour. In a different dish, beat the eggs. In a third shallow dish, add remaining ingredients except for fish fillets and mix till a crumbly mixture form.

Coat the fillets with flour and shake off the excess flour.

Dip the fillets in the egg.

Then coat the fillets with sesame seeds mixture generously.

Preheat the air fryer oven to 390 degrees F.

Line an Air fryer rack/basket with a piece of foil.

Arrange the fillets into the prepared basket.

Cook for about 14 minutes, flipping once after 10 minutes.

Nutrition:

Calories: 70
Carbs: 7g
Fat: 4g
Protein: 9g

311. Crispy Paprika Fish Fillets

Preparation time: 5 minutes
Cooking time: 15 minutes
Servings: 4

Ingredients:

1/2 cup seasoned breadcrumbs
1 tablespoon balsamic vinegar
1/2 teaspoon seasoned salt
1 teaspoon paprika
1/2 teaspoon ground black pepper
1 teaspoon celery seed
2 fish fillets, halved
1 egg, beaten

Directions:

Add the breadcrumbs, vinegar, salt, paprika, ground black pepper, and celery seeds to your food processor. Process for about 30 seconds.

Coat your fish fillets using the beaten egg; then, coat them with the breadcrumb's mixture.

Cook at 350 degrees F within 15 minutes.

Nutrition:

Calories: 140
Carbs: 9g
Fat: 7g
Protein: 5g

312.4-Ingredient Air Fryer Catfish

Preparation time: 5 minutes
Cooking time: 14 minutes
Servings: 4

Ingredients:

1 tbsp. chopped parsley

1 tbsp. olive oil
¼ C. seasoned fish fry
4 catfish fillets

Directions:

Ensure your Air Fryer Oven is preheated to 400 degrees.
Rinse off catfish fillets and pat dry.
Add fish fry seasoning to Ziploc baggie, then catfish. Shake the bag and ensure fish gets well coated.
Spray each fillet with olive oil. Add fillets to the air fryer basket.
Set temperature to 400°F, and set time to 10 minutes.
Cook 10 minutes. Then flip and cook another 2-3 minutes.

Nutrition:

Calories: 81
Carbs: 0g
Fat: 2g
Protein: 16g

313. Tuna Veggie Stir-Fry

Preparation time: 15 minutes
Cooking time: 12 minutes
Servings: 4

Ingredients:

1 tablespoon olive oil
1 red bell pepper, chopped
1 cup green beans
1 onion, sliced
2 cloves garlic, sliced
2 tablespoons low-sodium soy sauce
1 tablespoon honey
½ pound fresh tuna, cubed

Directions:

In a 6-inch metal bowl, combine the olive oil, pepper, green beans, onion, and garlic.
Set temperature to 350°F, and set time to 4 to 6 minutes, stirring once, until crisp and tender. Add soy sauce, honey, and tuna, and stir.
Cook for another 3 to 6 minutes, stirring once until the tuna is cooked as desired. Tuna can be served rare or medium-rare, or you can cook it until well done.

Nutrition:

Calories: 205
Carbs: 28g
Fat: 1g
Protein: 22g

314. Salmon Quiche

Preparation time: 15 minutes
Cooking time: 12 minutes
Servings: 4

Ingredients:

5 oz. Salmon Fillet
1/2 Tbsp Lemon Juice
1/2 Cup Flour
1/4 Cup Butter, melted
2 Eggs and 1 Egg Yolk
3 tbsp Whipped Cream
2 tbsp Mustard
Black Pepper to taste
Salt and Pepper
Quiche Pan

Directions:

Heat the Air Fryer Oven to 375 degrees
Pour the lemon juice over the salmon cubes and allow them to marinate for an hour.
Combine a tablespoon of water with the butter, flour, and yolk in a large bowl. Using your hands, knead the mixture until smooth
Use a rolling pin to form a circle of dough on a clean surface. Place this into the quiche pan, using your fingers to adhere the pastry to the edges
Whisk the cream, mustard, and eggs. Season with salt and pepper. Add the marinated salmon into the bowl and combine.
Pour the content of the bowl into the dough-lined quiche pan
Put the pan in the Air Fryer Oven tray and cook for 25 minutes until browned and crispy.

Nutrition:

Calories: 154
Carbs: 2g
Fat: 9g
Protein: 11g

315. Bang Panko Breaded Fried Shrimp

Preparation time: 5 minutes
Cooking time: 8 minutes
Servings: 4

Ingredients:

1 tsp. paprika
Montreal chicken seasoning
¾ C. panko bread crumbs
½ C. almond flour
1 egg white
1-pound raw shrimp (peeled and deveined)
Bang-Bang Sauce:
¼ C. sweet chili sauce
2 tbsp. sriracha sauce
1/3 C. plain Greek yogurt

Directions:

Ensure your Air Fryer Oven is preheated to 400 degrees.
Season all shrimp with seasonings.
Add flour to one bowl, egg white in another, and breadcrumbs to a third.
Dip seasoned shrimp in flour, then egg whites, and then breadcrumbs.
Spray coated shrimp with olive oil and add to the air fryer basket.
Set temperature to 400°F, and set time to 4 minutes.
Cook 4 minutes, flip, and cook an additional 4 minutes.
To make the sauce, mix all sauce ingredients until smooth.

Nutrition:

Calories: 190
Carbs: 18g
Fat: 8g
Protein: 12g

316. Flying Fish

Preparation time: 15 minutes
Cooking time: 12 minutes
Servings: 6

Ingredients:

4 tbsp Oil
3-4 oz Breadcrumbs
1 Whisked Whole Egg in a Saucer/Soup Plate
4 Fresh Fish Fillets
Fresh Lemon (For serving)

Directions:

Warm the air fryer to 350° F. Mix the crumbs and oil until it looks nice and loose.
Dip the fish in the egg and coat lightly, then move on to the crumbs. Make sure the fillet is covered evenly.
Cook in the Air Fryer Oven basket for roughly 12 minutes - depending on the size of the fillets you are using.
Serve with fresh lemon & chips to complete the duo.

Nutrition:

Calories: 211
Carbs: 0g
Fat: 2g
Protein: 46g

317. Pistachio-Crusted Lemon-Garlic Salmon

Preparation time: 15 minutes
Cooking time: 20 minutes
Servings: 6

Ingredients:

4 medium-sized salmon filets
2 raw eggs
3 ounces of melted butter
1 clove of garlic, minced
1 large-sized lemon
1 teaspoon of salt
1 tablespoon of parsley, rinsed, patted dry, and chopped
1 teaspoon of dill, rinsed, patted dry, and chopped
½ cup of pistachio nuts shelled and coarsely crushed

Directions:

Cover the air fryer basket with a lining of tin foil, leaving the edges uncovered to allow air to circulate through the basket.
Preheat the Air Fryer Oven to 350 degrees.
Whisk the eggs in a large mixing bowl.
Add the melted butter, the lemon's juice, the minced garlic, the parsley, and the dill to the beaten eggs and stir thoroughly.
One by one, dunk the salmon filets into the wet mixture, roll them in the crushed pistachios, coating completely.
Place the coated salmon fillets in the Air Fryer Oven basket.
Set the Air Fryer Oven timer for 10 minutes.
After 10 minutes, the salmon will be partially cooked when the air fryer shuts off, and the crust begins to crisp. Using tongs, turn each of the fish filets over.
Reset the Air Fryer Oven to 350 degrees for another 10 minutes.
After 10 minutes, when the air fryer shuts off, the salmon will be perfectly cooked, and the pistachio crust will be toasted and crispy. Using tongs, remove from the air fryer, and serve.

Nutrition:

Calories: 290
Carbs: 16g
Fat: 15g
Protein: 23g

318. Louisiana Shrimp Po Boy

Preparation time: 15 minutes
Cooking time: 10 minutes
Servings: 6

Ingredients:

1 tsp. creole seasoning
8 slices of tomato
Lettuce leaves
¼ C. buttermilk
½ C. Louisiana Fish Fry
1-pound deveined shrimp
Remoulade sauce:
1 chopped green onion
1 tsp. hot sauce
1 tsp. Dijon mustard
½ tsp. creole seasoning
1 tsp. Worcestershire sauce
Juice of ½ a lemon
½ C. vegan mayo

Directions:

Mix all sauce ingredients until well incorporated to make the sauce. Chill while you cook shrimp.
Mix seasonings and liberally season shrimp.
Add buttermilk to a bowl. Dip each shrimp into milk and place it in a Ziploc bag. Chill half an hour to marinate.
Add fish fry to a bowl. Take shrimp from the marinating bag and dip into fish fry, then add to the air fryer.
Ensure your air fryer is preheated to 400 degrees—spray shrimp with olive oil.
Set temperature to 400°F, and set time to 5 minutes. Cook 5 minutes, flip, and then cook another 5 minutes. Assemble "Keto" Po Boy by adding sauce to lettuce leaves, along with shrimp and tomato.

Nutrition:

Calories: 730
Carbs: 87g
Fat: 33g
Protein: 21g

319. Salmon Noodles

Preparation time: 5 minutes
Cooking time: 16 minutes
Servings: 4

Ingredients:

1 Salmon Fillet
1 Tbsp Teriyaki Marinade
3 ½ oz Soba Noodles, cooked and drained
10 oz Firm Tofu
7 oz Mixed Salad
1 cup Broccoli
Olive Oil
Salt and pepper to taste

Directions:

Massage the salmon with salt plus pepper to taste, then coat with the teriyaki marinade. Set aside for 15 minutes
Preheat the Air Fryer Oven to 350 degrees, then cook the salmon for 8 minutes.
While the air fryer is cooking the salmon, start slicing the tofu into small cubes.

Slice the broccoli into smaller chunks. Drizzle with olive oil.
Once the salmon is cooked, put the broccoli and tofu into the Air Fryer Oven tray for 8 minutes.
Plate the salmon and broccoli tofu mixture over the soba noodles. Add the mixed salad to the side and serve.

Nutrition:

Calories: 650
Carbs: 45g
Fat: 5g
Protein: 4g

320. Beer-Battered Fish and Chips

Preparation time: 15 minutes
Cooking time: 30 minutes
Servings: 4

Ingredients:

2 eggs
1 cup malty beer, such as Pabst Blue Ribbon
1 cup all-purpose flour
½ cup cornstarch
1 teaspoon garlic powder
Salt
Pepper
Cooking oil
(4-ounce) cod fillets

Directions:

Whisk the eggs with the beer in a medium bowl. In another medium bowl, combine the flour and cornstarch and season with the garlic powder and salt and pepper to taste.
Grease the air fryer basket with cooking oil.
Dip each cod fillet in the flour and cornstarch mixture and then in the egg and beer mixture. Dip the cod in the flour and cornstarch a second time.
Place the cod in the Air Fryer Oven. Do not stack—Cook in batches. Spray with cooking oil—Cook for 8 minutes.
Open the Air Fryer Oven and flip the cod. Cook for an additional 7 minutes.
Remove the cooked cod from the air fryer, repeat steps 4 and 5 for the remaining fillets.
Serve with prepared air-fried frozen fries. Frozen fries will need to be cooked for 18 to 20 minutes at 400ºF.
Cool before serving.

Nutrition:

Calories: 398
Carbs: 41g
Fat: 15g
Protein: 25g

321. Tuna Stuffed Potatoes

Preparation time: 15 minutes
Cooking time: 30 minutes
Servings: 4

Ingredients:

4 starchy potatoes
½ tablespoon olive oil
1 can tuna, drained
2 tablespoons plain Greek yogurt
1 teaspoon red chili powder
Salt
ground black pepper
1 scallion, chopped and divided
1 tablespoon capers

Directions:

Submerged the potatoes for about 30 minutes in a large bowl of water. Drain well and pat dry with a paper towel.
Preheat the air fryer to 355 degrees F. Place the potatoes in a fryer basket.
Cook for about 30 minutes.
Meanwhile, in a bowl, add tuna, yogurt, red chili powder, salt, black pepper, and half of the scallion, and with a potato masher, mash the mixture thoroughly.
Remove the potatoes from the Air Fryer Oven and place it onto a smooth surface.
Carefully cut each potato from the top side lengthwise.
With your fingers, press the open side of potato halves slightly. Stuff the open potato portion with tuna mixture evenly.
Sprinkle with the capers and remaining scallion. Serve immediately.

Nutrition:

Calories: 344
Carbs: 44g
Fat: 8g
Protein: 26g

322. Potato Crusted Salmon

Preparation time: 15 minutes
Cooking time: 15 minutes
Servings: 4

Ingredients:

1-pound salmon, swordfish, or arctic char fillets, 3/4 inch thick
1 egg white
2 tablespoons water
1/3 cup dry instant mashed potatoes
2 teaspoons cornstarch
1 teaspoon paprika
1 teaspoon lemon pepper seasoning

Directions:

Remove and skin from the fish and cut it into 4 serving pieces. Mix the egg white and water. Mix all of the dry ingredients. Dip the fillets into the egg white mixture, then press into the potato mix to coat evenly.
Put it on the air fryer basket. Set temperature to 360°F, and set time to 15 minutes, flip the filets halfway through.

Nutrition:

Calories: 315
Carbs: 14g
Fat: 18g
Protein: 24g

323. Salmon Croquettes

Preparation time: 15 minutes
Cooking time: 10 minutes
Servings: 8

Ingredients:

Panko breadcrumbs
Almond flour

2 egg whites
2 tbsp. chopped chives
2 tbsp. minced garlic cloves
½ C. chopped onion
2/3 C. grated carrots
1-pound chopped salmon fillet

Directions:

Mix all ingredients minus breadcrumbs, flour, and egg whites.
Shape mixture into balls. Then coat them in flour, then egg, and then breadcrumbs. Drizzle with olive oil.
Pour the coated salmon balls into the oven rack. Place it on the middle-shelf position of the Air Fryer Oven. Set temperature to 350°F, and set time to 6 minutes. Shake and cook an additional 4 minutes until golden in color.

Nutrition:

Calories: 192
Carbs: 0g
Fat: 10g
Protein: 25g

324. Snapper Scampi

Preparation time: 15 minutes
Cooking time: 10 minutes
Servings: 4

Ingredients:

4 (6-ounce) skinless snapper or arctic char fillets
1 tablespoon olive oil
3 tablespoons lemon juice, divided
½ teaspoon dried basil
Pinch salt
Freshly ground black pepper
2 tablespoons butter
cloves garlic, minced

Directions:

Massage the fish fillets with olive oil and 1 tablespoon of the lemon juice. Sprinkle with the basil, salt, and pepper, and place in the Air Fryer Oven basket.
Grill the fish for 7 to 8 minutes or until the fish just flakes when tested with a fork. Remove the fish from the basket and put on a serving plate.
Cover to keep warm. In a 6-by-6-by-2-inch pan, combine the butter, remaining 2 tablespoons lemon juice, and garlic.
Cook in the Air Fryer Oven for 1 to 2 minutes or until the garlic is sizzling. Pour this mixture over the fish and serve.

Nutrition:

Calories: 540
Carbs: 0g
Fat: 12g
Protein: 0g

325. Air Fryer Fish Tacos

Preparation time: 15 minutes
Cooking time: 15 minutes
Servings: 4

Ingredients:

1-pound cod
1 tbsp. cumin
½ tbsp. chili powder
1 ½ C. almond flour
1 ½ C. coconut flour
10 ounces Mexican beer
2 eggs

Directions:

Whisk beer and eggs in a bowl.
Whisk flours, pepper, salt, cumin, and chili powder in a separate bowl.
Slice cod into large pieces and coat in egg mixture then flour mixture.
Spray the bottom of your Air Fryer Oven basket with olive oil and add coated codpieces. Cook 15 minutes at 375 degrees.
Serve on lettuce leaves topped with homemade salsa.

Nutrition:

Calories: 117
Carbs: 2g
Fat: 6g
Protein: 12g

326. Bacon-Wrapped Scallops

Preparation time: 15 minutes
Cooking time: 5 minutes
Servings: 4

Ingredients:

1 tsp. paprika
1 tsp. lemon pepper
5 slices of center-cut bacon
20 raw sea scallops

Directions:

Rinse and drain scallops, placing on paper towels to soak up excess moisture.
Cut slices of bacon into 4 pieces.
Wrap the scallop with the bacon, using toothpicks to secure. Sprinkle wrapped scallops with paprika and lemon pepper.
Spray the air fryer basket using olive oil and add scallops.
Cook 5-6 minutes at 400 degrees, making sure to flip halfway through.

Nutrition:

Calories: 270
Carbs: 1g
Fat: 24g
Protein: 12g

327. Delicious Cajun Salmon

Preparation time: 15 minutes
Cooking time: 12 minutes
Servings: 2

Ingredients:

4 salmon fillets
4 tbsp brown sugar
2 tsp Cajun seasoning
Salt

Directions:

Mix Cajun seasoning, brown sugar, and salt and rub all over salmon.
Place salmon on the baking pan. Set to Convection Bake at 400°F for 12 minutes.
Serve and enjoy.

Nutrition:

Calories 271
Fat 10 g

Carbohydrates 8 g
Sugar 8 g
Protein 34 g

328. Flavors Lemon Cod

Preparation time: 15 minutes
Cooking time: 20 minutes
Servings: 4
Ingredients:
1 1/2 lb. cod fillet
2 lemon juice
2 tbsp olive oil
1 lemon, sliced
1/4 cup butter, diced
4 garlic cloves, minced
Pepper
Salt
Directions:
Place fish fillets in the baking pan and season with pepper and salt.
Whisk garlic, lemon juice, and oil and pour over fish fillets.
Arrange butter pieces and lemon slices on top of fish fillets.
Set to "Convection Bake" at 400°F for 20 minutes.
Serve and enjoy.
Nutrition:
Calories 309
Fat 20 g
Carbohydrates 2 g
Sugar 0.6 g
Protein 31 g

329. Spicy Tilapia

Preparation time: 15 minutes
Cooking time: 15 minutes
Servings: 4
Ingredients:
4 tilapia fillets
1/2 tsp red chili powder
1 tsp garlic, minced
3 tbsp butter, melted
1 tbsp fresh lemon juice
2 tsp fresh parsley, chopped
1 lemon, sliced
Pepper
Salt
Directions:
Place fish fillets in the foiled baking pan and season with pepper and salt.
Mix butter, red chili powder, garlic, and lemon juice and pour over fish fillets.
Arrange lemon slices on top of fish fillets.
Set to Convection Bake at 350°F for 15 minutes.
Garnish with parsley and serve.
Nutrition:
Calories 149
Fat 12 g
Carbohydrates 4 g
Sugar 0.1 g
Protein 6 g
Cholesterol 38 mg

330. Garlic Lime Shrimp

Preparation time: 15 minutes
Cooking time: 15 minutes
Servings: 4
Ingredients:
1 lb. shrimp, peel and deveined
2 tbsp lime juice
2 tbsp butter, melted
1/4 cup fresh cilantro, chopped
3 garlic cloves, pressed
Directions:
Add shrimp into the baking dish.
Mix garlic, lime juice, and butter and pour over shrimp.
Toss shrimp well and let it sit for 15 minutes.
Set to Convection Bake at 375°F for 15 minutes.
Garnish with cilantro and serve.
Nutrition:
Calories 195
Fat 7.7 g
Carbohydrates 4.4 g
Sugar 0.4 g
Protein 26.1 g

331. Dijon Salmon

Preparation time: 15 minutes
Cooking time: 12 minutes
Servings: 4
Ingredients:
4 salmon fillets
1/4 cup Dijon mustard
1/4 cup maple syrup
2 garlic cloves, minced
2 tbsp olive oil
Pepper
Salt
Directions:
Place salmon fillets into the baking pan.
Mix garlic, olive oil, Dijon mustard, maple syrup, pepper, salt, and pour over salmon. Coat, then let sit for 10 minutes.
Set to "Bake" at 400°F for 12 minutes. Serve and enjoy.
Nutrition:
Calories 360
Fat 18 g
Carbohydrates 14 g
Sugar 12 g
Protein 35 g

332. Parmesan Walnut Salmon

Preparation time: 15 minutes
Cooking time: 15 minutes
Servings: 4
Ingredients:
4 salmon fillets
1/4 cup walnuts
1 tsp olive oil
1/4 cup parmesan cheese, grated
1 tbsp lemon rind
Directions:
Place salmon fillets in the baking pan.
Add walnuts into the blender and blend until ground.
Mix the walnuts, cheese, oil, and lemon rind and spread on top of salmon fillets.

Bake at 400°F for 15 minutes. Serve and enjoy.
Nutrition:
Calories 312
Fat 18 g
Carbohydrates 1 g
Sugar 0.2 g
Protein 38 g

333. Greek Pesto Salmon

Preparation time: 15 minutes
Cooking time: 20 minutes
Servings: 4
Ingredients:
4 salmon fillets
1/2 cup pesto
1/2 cup feta cheese, crumbled
2 cups grape tomatoes, halved
1 onion, chopped
Directions:
Place salmon fillet in the baking pan with foil and top with tomatoes, onion, pesto, and cheese.
Set to Convection Bake at 350°F for 20 minutes.
Serve and enjoy.
Nutrition:
Calories 447
Fat 28 g
Carbohydrates 8 g
Sugar 6 g
Protein 41 g

334. Easy Baked Tilapia

Preparation time: 15 minutes
Cooking time: 15 minutes
Servings: 4
Ingredients:
1 lb. tilapia fillets
2 tbsp garlic, minced
2 tbsp olive oil
2 tbsp dried parsley
Pepper
Salt
Directions:
Place fish fillets on a baking pan with foil. Drizzle with oil and season with pepper and salt.
Sprinkle garlic and parsley over fish fillets.
Set to "Bake" at 400°F for 15 minutes. Serve and enjoy.
Nutrition:
Calories 160
Fat 8 g
Carbohydrates 1 g
Sugar 0.1 g
Protein 21 g

335. Cajun Catfish Fillets

Preparation time: 15 minutes
Cooking time: 15 minutes
Servings: 4
Ingredients:
1 lb. catfish fillets, cut ½-inch thick
1/2 tsp ground cumin
3/4 tsp chili powder
1 tsp crushed red pepper
2 tsp onion powder
1 tbsp dried oregano, crushed
Pepper
Salt
Directions:
Mix cumin, chili powder, crushed red pepper, onion powder, oregano, pepper, and salt in a small bowl.
Rub fish fillets with the spice mixture on both sides.
Place fish fillets in a baking pan.
Set to Bake at 350°F for 15 minutes. Serve and enjoy.
Nutrition:
Calories 165
Fat 9 g
Carbohydrates 2 g
Sugar 0.6 g
Protein 18 g
Cholesterol 53 mg

336. Blackened Mahi-Mahi

Preparation time: 15 minutes
Cooking time: 12 minutes
Servings: 4
Ingredients:
4 Mahi-Mahi fillets
1 tsp paprika
1 tsp garlic powder
3 tbsp Olive oil
1/2 cayenne
1 tsp oregano
1 tsp cumin
1 tsp onion powder
1/2 tsp pepper
1/2 tsp salt
Directions:
Place fish fillets on the baking pan and drizzle with oil.
In a small bowl, mix cumin, onion powder, paprika, cayenne, oregano, garlic powder, pepper, and salt.
Rub fish fillets with a spice mixture.
Set to Convection Bake at 450°F for 12 minutes.
Serve and enjoy.
Nutrition:
Calories 189
Fat 12 g
Carbohydrates 2 g
Sugar 0.5 g
Protein 19 g

337. Salmon Dill Patties

Preparation time: 15 minutes
Cooking time: 10 minutes
Servings: 2
Ingredients:
1 egg
1 tsp dill weed
1/2 cup almond flour
14 oz salmon
1/4 cup onion, diced
Directions:
Add all fixing into the bowl and mix well.
Make patties from bowl mixture and place onto the air fryer basket.
Set to air fry at 375°F for 10 minutes.
Serve and enjoy.
Nutrition:

Calories 350
Fat 18 g
Carbohydrates 3 g
Sugar 1 g
Protein 44 g

338. Spicy Shrimp

Preparation time: 15 minutes
Cooking time: 6 minutes
Servings: 2

Ingredients:

1/2 lb. shrimp, peeled and deveined
1/2 tsp old bay seasoning
1/2 tsp cayenne pepper
1 tbsp olive oil
1/4 tsp paprika
Pinch of salt

Directions:

Add shrimp and remaining ingredients into the bowl and toss well to coat.
Add shrimp into the greased air fryer basket.
Set to air fry at 400°F for 6 minutes. Serve and enjoy.

Nutrition:

Calories 197
Fat 9 g
Carbohydrates 2 g
Sugar 0.1 g
Protein 26 g
Cholesterol 239 mg

339. White Fish Fillet

Preparation time: 15 minutes
Cooking time: 10 minutes
Servings: 2

Ingredients:

12 oz white fish fillets
1/2 tsp lemon pepper seasoning
1/2 tsp garlic powder
1/2 tsp onion powder
Pepper
Salt

Directions:

Spray fish fillets with cooking spray and season with onion powder, lemon pepper seasoning, garlic powder, pepper, and salt.
Place parchment paper in the bottom of the air fryer basket. Place fish fillets into the air fryer basket.
Set to air fry at 350°F for 10 minutes. Serve and enjoy.

Nutrition:

Calories 298
Fat 13 g
Carbohydrates 1.4 g
Sugar 0.4 g
Protein 42 g

340. Coconut Shrimp

Preparation time: 15 minutes
Cooking time:
minutes
Servings: 8

Ingredients:

2 eggs, lightly beaten
1 lb. large shrimp, peeled and deveined
1 cup flaked coconut
1/4 cup coconut flour

Directions:

In a small bowl, add coconut flour.
In a shallow bowl, add eggs. In a separate shallow bowl, add flaked coconut.
Coat shrimp with coconut flour, then dip in eggs and finally coat with flaked coconut.
Place coated shrimp into the air fryer basket.
Set to air fry at 400°F for 8 minutes. Serve and enjoy.

Nutrition:

Calories 112
Fat 5 g
Carbohydrates 5 g
Sugar 0.7 g
Protein 13 g

341. Parmesan Fish Fillets

Preparation time: 15 minutes
Cooking time: 10 minutes
Servings: 4

Ingredients:

1 lb. white fish fillets
1/2 tsp lemon pepper seasoning
1/4 cup coconut flour
1/4 cup parmesan cheese

Directions:

In a shallow dish, mix coconut flour, parmesan cheese, and lemon pepper seasoning.
Spray white fish fillets from both sides with cooking spray.
Coat fish fillets with coconut flour mixture. Place coated fish fillets into the air fryer basket.
Set to air fry at 400°F for 10 minutes. Serve and enjoy.

Nutrition:

Calories 220
Fat 10 g
Carbohydrates 1 g
Sugar 0.1 g
Protein 30 g

Chapter 8. Vegetables

342. Lemony Wax Beans

Preparation time: 5 minutes
Cooking time: 12 minutes
Servings: 4
Ingredients:
2 pounds (907 g) wax beans
2 tablespoons extra-virgin olive oil
Salt
ground black pepper
Juice of ½ lemon, for serving
Directions:
Line a baking sheet with aluminum foil.
Toss the wax beans with the olive oil in a large bowl. Lightly season with salt and pepper.
Spread out the wax beans on the sheet pan.
Select Roast, set temperature to 400ºF (205ºC), and set time to 12 minutes.
Once preheated, place the baking sheet into the oven.
When done, the beans will be caramelized and tender.
Serve sprinkled with the lemon juice.
Nutrition:
Calories: 44
Carbs: 6g
Fat: 0g
Protein: 2g

343. Lemony Brussels Sprouts and Tomatoes

Preparation time: 15 minutes
Cooking time: 20 minutes
Servings: 4
Ingredients:
1-pound (454 g) Brussels sprouts, trimmed and halved
1 tablespoon extra-virgin olive oil
Sea Salt
ground black pepper
½ cup sun-dried tomatoes, chopped
2 tablespoons freshly squeezed lemon juice
1 teaspoon lemon zest
Directions:
Line a large baking sheet with aluminum foil.
Toss the Brussels sprouts with the olive oil in a large bowl. Sprinkle with salt and black pepper.
Arrange the brussels sprouts on the baking sheet.
Select Roast, set temperature to 400ºF (205ºC), and set time to 20 minutes.
Once preheated, place the baking sheet into the oven.
When done, the Brussels sprouts should be caramelized. Transfer to a serving bowl, along with the tomatoes, lemon juice, and lemon zest. Toss to combine. Serve immediately.
Nutrition:
Calories: 70
Carbs: 11g
Fat: 3g
Protein: 3g

344. Maple and Pecan Granola

Preparation time: 5 minutes
Cooking time: 20 minutes
Servings: 4
Ingredients:
1½ cups rolled oats
¼ cup maple syrup
¼ cup pecan pieces
1 teaspoon vanilla extract
½ teaspoon ground cinnamon
Directions:
Line a baking sheet with parchment paper.
Mix the oats, maple syrup, pecan pieces, vanilla, and cinnamon in a large bowl and stir until the oats and pecan pieces are completely coated. Spread the batter on the baking sheet.
Set temperature to 300ºF (150ºC), and set time to 20 minutes.
Once preheated, place the baking sheet into the oven.
Stir once halfway through the cooking time.
When done, cool it for 30 minutes before serving.
The granola may still be a bit soft right after removing, but it will gradually firm up as it cools.
Nutrition:
Calories: 137
Carbs: 18g
Fat: 6g
Protein: 3g

345. Sweet and Spicy Broccoli

Preparation time: 10 minutes
Cooking time: 20 minutes
Servings: 4
Ingredients:
½ teaspoon olive oil, plus more for greasing
1 pound (454 g) fresh broccoli, cut into florets
½ tablespoon minced garlic
Salt, to taste
Sauce:
1½ tablespoons soy sauce
2 teaspoons hot sauce or sriracha
1½ teaspoons honey
1 teaspoon white vinegar
Freshly ground black pepper, to taste
Directions:
Grease a perforated pan with olive oil.
Add the broccoli florets, ½ teaspoon of olive oil, and garlic to a large bowl and toss well—season with salt to taste.
Put the broccoli in the perforated pan in a single layer.
Select Air Fry, set temperature to 400ºF (205ºC), and set time to 15 minutes.
Once preheated, place the pan into the oven. Stir the broccoli florets three times during cooking.
Meanwhile, whisk all the ingredients for the sauce in a small bowl until well incorporated.
The broccoli should be lightly browned and crispy.
Continue cooking for 5 minutes, if desired. Transfer and pour over the sauce and toss to combine. Add more salt and pepper if needed. Serve warm.
Nutrition:
Calories: 68
Carbs: 4g
Fat: 4g

Protein: 3g

346. Roasted Vegetables with Basil

Preparation time: 15 minutes
Cooking time: 20 minutes
Servings: 2

Ingredients:

1 small eggplant, halved and sliced
1 yellow bell pepper, strips
1 red bell pepper, strips
2 garlic cloves, quartered
1 red onion, sliced
1 tablespoon extra-virgin olive oil
Salt
ground black pepper
½ cup chopped fresh basil, for garnish
Cooking spray

Directions:

Grease a nonstick baking dish with cooking spray.
Place the eggplant, bell peppers, garlic, and red onion in the greased baking dish. Drizzle with the olive oil and toss to coat well. Spritz any uncoated surfaces with cooking spray.
Set temperature to 350ºF (180ºC), and set time to 20 minutes.
Turn over the vegetables halfway through the cooking time. When done, put salt plus pepper.
Sprinkle the basil on top for garnish and serve.

Nutrition:

Calories: 60
Carbs: 8g
Fat: 3g
Protein: 1g

347. Cinnamon Celery Roots

Preparation time: 10 minutes
Cooking time: 20 minutes
Servings: 4

Ingredients:

2 celery roots, peeled and diced
1 teaspoon extra-virgin olive oil
1 teaspoon butter, melted
½ teaspoon ground cinnamon
Sea salt
ground black pepper

Directions:

Line a baking sheet with aluminum foil.
Toss the celery roots with the olive oil in a large bowl until well coated. Transfer them to the prepared baking sheet.
Select Roast, set temperature to 350ºF (180ºC), and set time to 20 minutes.
When done, the celery roots should be very tender.
Transfer, then stir in the butter and cinnamon and mash them with a potato masher until fluffy.
Season with salt and pepper to taste. Serve immediately.

Nutrition:

Calories: 36
Carbs: 8g
Fat: 0g
Protein: 0g

348. Cheesy Broccoli Tots

Preparation time: 20 minutes
Cooking time: 15 minutes
Servings: 4

Ingredients:

12 ounces (340 g) frozen broccoli, thawed, drained, and patted dry
1 large egg, lightly beaten
½ cup seasoned whole-wheat bread crumbs
¼ cup shredded reduced-fat sharp Cheddar cheese
¼ cup grated Parmesan cheese
1½ teaspoons minced garlic
Salt
ground black pepper
Cooking spray

Directions:

Spritz a perforated pan lightly with cooking spray.
Place the remaining ingredients into a food processor and process until the mixture resembles a coarse meal. Transfer the mixture to a bowl.
Using a tablespoon, scoop out the broccoli mixture and form into 24 oval "tater tot" shapes with your hands.
Put the tots in the prepared perforated pan in a single layer, spacing them 1 inch apart. Mist the tots lightly with cooking spray.
Select Air Fry, set temperature to 375ºF (190ºC), and set time to 15 minutes.
Flip the tots halfway through the cooking time.
When done, the tots will be lightly browned and crispy. Serve on a plate.

Nutrition:

Calories: 12
Carbs: 2g
Fat: 3g
Protein: 4g

349. Paprika Cauliflower

Preparation time: 10 minutes
Cooking time: 20 minutes
Servings: 4

Ingredients:

1 large head cauliflower, florets
2 teaspoons smoked paprika
1 teaspoon garlic powder
Salt
ground black pepper
Cooking spray

Directions:

Spray a perforated pan with cooking spray.
Toss the cauliflower florets with the smoked paprika and garlic powder until evenly coated in a medium bowl. Sprinkle with salt and pepper.
Place the cauliflower florets in the perforated pan and lightly mist with cooking spray.
Select Air Fry, set temperature to 400ºF (205ºC), and set time to 20 minutes.
Stir the cauliflower four times during cooking.
Remove and serve hot.

Nutrition:

Calories: 90
Carbs: 4g
Fat: 8g
Protein: 2g

350. Roasted Asparagus with Eggs and Tomatoes

Preparation time: 10 minutes
Cooking time: 12 minutes
Servings: 4

Ingredients:

2 pounds (907 g) asparagus, trimmed
3 tablespoons extra-virgin olive oil, divided
1 teaspoon kosher salt, divided
1-pint cherry tomatoes
4 large eggs
¼ teaspoon freshly ground black pepper

Directions:

Put the asparagus on the sheet pan and drizzle with 2 tablespoons of olive oil, tossing to coat. Season with ½ teaspoon of kosher salt.
Select Roast, set temperature to 375ºF (190ºC), and cook within 12 minutes.
Meanwhile, toss the cherry tomatoes with the remaining 1 tablespoon of olive oil in a medium bowl until well coated.
After 6 minutes, remove the pan and toss the asparagus. Evenly spread the asparagus in the middle of the sheet pan. Add the tomatoes around the perimeter of the pan. Return it to the oven.
After 2 minutes, remove the pan from the oven. Carefully crack the eggs, one at a time, over the asparagus, spacing them out—season with the remaining ½ teaspoon of kosher salt and the pepper. Return it to the oven, then cook for an additional 3 to 7 minutes.
When done, divide the asparagus and eggs among four plates. Top each plate evenly with the tomatoes and serve.

Nutrition:

Calories: 335
Carbs: 0g
Fat: 0g
Protein: 0g

351. Ratatouille

Preparation time: 10 minutes
Cooking time: 12 minutes
Servings: 6

Ingredients:

1 medium zucchini, sliced ½-inch thick
1 small eggplant, peeled and sliced ½-inch thick
2 teaspoons kosher salt, divided
4 tablespoons extra-virgin olive oil, divided
3 garlic cloves, minced
1 small onion, chopped
1 small red bell pepper, cut into ½-inch chunks
1 small green bell pepper, cut into ½-inch chunks
½ teaspoon dried oregano
¼ teaspoon freshly ground black pepper
1-pint cherry tomatoes
2 tablespoons minced fresh basil
1 cup panko bread crumbs
½ cup grated Parmesan cheese (optional)

Directions:

Season one side of the zucchini and eggplant slices with ¾ teaspoon of salt. Put the slices, salted side down, on a rack set over a baking sheet. Sprinkle the other sides with ¾ teaspoon of salt.
Allow to sit for 10 minutes, or until the slices begin to exude water. When ready, rinse and dry them. Cut the zucchini slices into quarters, and the eggplant slices into eighths.
Pour the zucchini and eggplant into a large bowl, along with 2 tablespoons of olive oil, garlic, onion, bell peppers, oregano, and black pepper. Toss to coat well. Arrange the vegetables on the sheet pan.
Select Roast, set temperature to 375ºF (190ºC), and cook within 12 minutes.
At the same time, mix the tomatoes and basil to the large bowl. Sprinkle with the remaining ½ teaspoon of salt and 1 tablespoon of olive oil. Toss well and set aside.
Stir the remaining 1 tablespoon of olive oil, panko, and Parmesan cheese (if desired) in a small bowl.
After 6 minutes, remove the pan, add the tomato mixture to the sheet pan, and mix well. Scatter the panko mixture on top.
Return it and cook again within 6 minutes or until the vegetables are softened, and the topping is golden brown.
Cool for 5 minutes before serving.

Nutrition:

Calories: 189
Carbs: 15g
Fat: 12g
Protein: 3g

352. Bean, Salsa, and Cheese Tacos

Preparation time: 15 minutes
Cooking time: 7 minutes
Servings: 4

Ingredients:

1 can black beans, drained
½ cup prepared salsa
1½ teaspoons chili powder
4 ounces (113 g) grated Monterey Jack cheese
2 tablespoons minced onion
8 (6-inch) flour tortillas
2 tablespoons vegetable or extra-virgin olive oil
Shredded lettuce, for serving

Directions:

In a medium bowl, add the beans, salsa, and chili powder. Coarsely mash them with a potato masher. Fold in the cheese and onion and stir until combined.
Arrange the flour tortillas on a cutting board and spoon 2 to 3 tablespoons of the filling into each tortilla. Fold the tortillas over, pressing lightly to even out the filling. Brush the tacos on one side with half the olive oil and put them, oiled side down, on the sheet pan. Brush the top side with the remaining olive oil.
Select Air Fry, set temperature to 400ºF (205ºC), and set time to 7 minutes.
Flip the tacos halfway through the cooking time.
Remove, then allow to cool within 5 minutes. Serve with the shredded lettuce on the side.

Nutrition:

Calories: 220
Carbs: 24g
Fat: 10g

Protein: 10g

353. Spicy Thai-Style Vegetables

Preparation time: 10 minutes
Cooking time: 8 minutes
Servings: 4

Ingredients:

1 small head Napa cabbage, shredded, divided
1 medium carrot, cut into thin coins
8 ounces (227 g) snow peas
1 red or green bell pepper, strips
1 tablespoon vegetable oil
2 tablespoons soy sauce
1 tablespoon sesame oil
2 tablespoons brown sugar
2 tablespoons freshly squeezed lime juice
2 tsp red Thai curry paste
1 serrano Chile, deseeded and minced
1 cup frozen mango slices, thawed
½ cup chopped roasted peanuts or cashews

Directions:

Put half the Napa cabbage in a large bowl, along with the carrot, snow peas, and bell pepper. Drizzle with the vegetable oil and toss to coat. Spread them evenly on the sheet pan.
Select Roast, set temperature to 375ºF (190ºC), and set time to 8 minutes.
Meanwhile, whisk the soy sauce, sesame oil, brown sugar, lime juice, and curry paste in a small bowl.
When done, the vegetables should be tender and crisp. Remove the pan and put the vegetables back into the bowl. Add Chile, mango slices, and the remaining cabbage. Pour over the dressing and toss to coat. Top with the roasted nuts and serve.

Nutrition:

Calories: 35
Carbs: 8g
Fat: 0g
Protein: 2g

354. Balsamic Asparagus

Preparation time: 15 minutes
Cooking time: 10 minutes
Servings: 4

Ingredients:

4 tablespoons olive oil
4 tablespoons balsamic vinegar
1½ pounds (680 g) asparagus spears, trimmed
Salt
ground black pepper

Directions:

Grease a perforated pan with olive oil.
In a shallow bowl, stir the 4 tablespoons of olive oil and balsamic vinegar to make a marinade.
Put the asparagus spears in the bowl, so they are thoroughly covered by the marinade and allow to marinate for 5 minutes.
Put the asparagus in the greased perforated pan in a single layer and season with salt and pepper.
Select Air Fry, set temperature to 350ºF (180ºC), and set time to 10 minutes.
Flip the asparagus halfway through the cooking time.
When done, the asparagus should be tender and lightly browned. Cool for 5 minutes before serving.

Nutrition:

Calories: 90
Carbs: 0g
Fat: 5g
Protein: 4g

355. Tortellini with Veggies and Parmesan

Preparation time: 10 minutes
Cooking time: 16 minutes
Servings: 4

Ingredients:

8 ounces (227 g) sugar snap peas, trimmed
½ pound (227 g) asparagus, trimmed and cut into 1-inch pieces
2 teaspoons kosher salt or 1 teaspoon fine salt, divided
1 tablespoon extra-virgin olive oil
1½ cups water
1 (20-ounce / 340-g) package frozen cheese tortellini
2 garlic cloves, minced
1 cup heavy (whipping) cream
1 cup cherry tomatoes, halved
½ cup grated Parmesan cheese
¼ cup chopped fresh parsley or basil

Directions:

Add the peas and asparagus to a large bowl. Add ½ teaspoon of kosher salt and the olive oil and toss until well coated. Place the veggies in the sheet pan.
Set the temperature to 450ºF (235ºC), and set the time for 4 minutes.
Meanwhile, dissolve 1 teaspoon of kosher salt in the water.
Once cooking is complete, remove the pan from the oven and arrange the tortellini on the pan. Pour the salted water over the tortellini. Transfer the pan back to the oven.
Set temperature to 450ºF (235ºC), and set time for 7 minutes.
Meantime, stir the garlic, heavy cream, and remaining ½ teaspoon of kosher salt in a small bowl.
Once cooking is complete, remove the pan from the oven. Blot off any remaining water with a paper towel, then gently stir the ingredients. Drizzle the cream over and top with the tomatoes.
Select Roast, set the temperature to 375ºF (190ºC), and set the time for 5 minutes.
Put the Parmesan cheese and stir until the cheese is melted. Serve topped with the parsley.

Nutrition:

Calories: 290
Carbs: 31g
Fat: 10g
Protein: 17g

356. Mediterranean Baked Eggs with Spinach

Preparation time: 15 minutes
Cooking time: 10 minutes
Servings: 2

Ingredients:

2 tablespoons olive oil
4 eggs, whisked
5 ounces (142 g) fresh spinach, chopped
1 medium-sized tomato, chopped

1 teaspoon fresh lemon juice
½ teaspoon ground black pepper
½ teaspoon coarse salt
½ cup basil leaves, roughly chopped for garnish

Directions:

Grease your baking pan with olive oil.
Stir the remaining ingredients except for the basil leaves in the greased baking pan until well incorporated.
Set temperature to 280ºF (137ºC), and set time to 10 minutes.
The eggs should be set entirely, and the vegetables should be tender. Remove, then serve garnished with the fresh basil leaves.

Nutrition:

Calories: 170
Carbs: 1g
Fat: 9g
Protein: 7g

357. Sandwiches with Tomato, Nuts & Cheese

Preparation time: 30 minutes
Cooking time: 12 minutes
Servings: 2

Ingredients:

1 heirloom tomato
1 (4-oz) block feta cheese
1 small red onion, thinly sliced
1 clove garlic
Salt to taste
2 tsp + ¼ cup olive oil
1 ½ tbsp toasted pine nuts
¼ cup chopped parsley
¼ cup grated Parmesan cheese
¼ cup chopped basil

Directions:

Put the basil, pine nuts, garlic, plus salt to a food processor. Process while slowly adding ¼ cup of olive oil. Once finished, pour basil pesto into a bowl and refrigerate for 30 minutes.
Preheat on Air Fry function to 390 F. Slice the feta cheese and tomato into ½-inch slices. Remove the pesto from the fridge and spread half of it on the tomato slices. Top with feta cheese slices and onion. Drizzle the remaining olive oil on top.
Place the tomatoes in the fryer basket and fit in the baking tray; cook for 12 minutes. Remove to a serving platter and top with the remaining pesto. Serve.

Nutrition:

Calories: 208
Carbs: 1g
Fat: 12g
Protein: 3g

358. Vegetable Fried Mix Chips

Preparation time: 15 minutes
Cooking time: 12 minutes
Servings: 4

Ingredients:

1 large eggplant
4 potatoes
3 zucchinis
½ cup cornstarch
½ cup olive oil
Salt to season

Directions:

Preheat on Air Fry function to 390 F. Cut the eggplant and zucchini in long 3-inch strips. Peel and cut the potatoes into 3-inch strips; set aside.
In a bowl, stir in cornstarch, ½ cup of water, salt, pepper, oil, eggplant, zucchini, and potatoes. Place one-third of the veggie strips in the basket and fit in the baking tray; cook for 12 minutes, shaking once. Once ready, transfer them to a serving platter. Repeat the cooking process for the remaining veggie strips. Serve warm.

Nutrition:

Calories: 230
Carbs: 39g
Fat: 7g
Protein: 2g

359. Cayenne Spicy Green Beans

Preparation time: 15 minutes
Cooking time: 15 minutes
Servings: 4

Ingredients:

1 cup panko breadcrumbs
2 whole eggs, beaten
½ cup Parmesan cheese, grated
½ cup flour
1 tsp cayenne pepper
1 ½ pounds green beans
Salt to taste

Directions:

In a bowl, mix panko breadcrumbs, Parmesan cheese, cayenne pepper, salt, and pepper. Roll the green beans in flour and dip in eggs.
Dredge beans in the parmesan-panko mix. Place the prepared beans in the greased cooking basket and fit in the baking tray; cook for 15 minutes on Air Fry function at 350 F, shaking once.
Serve and enjoy!

Nutrition:

Calories: 50
Carbs: 9g
Fat: 2g
Protein: 2g

360. Cheesy Cabbage Wedges

Preparation time: 15 minutes
Cooking time: 20 minutes
Servings: 4

Ingredients:

½ head cabbage, cut into wedges
2 cups Parmesan cheese, chopped
4 tbsp melted butter
Salt and black pepper to taste
½ cup blue cheese sauce

Directions:

Brush the cabbage wedges with butter and coat with mozzarella cheese.
Place the coated wedges in the greased basket and fit in the baking tray; cook for 20 minutes at 380 F on the Air Fry setting. Serve with blue cheese sauce.

Nutrition:

Calories: 108
Carbs: 12g
Fat: 7g
Protein: 2g

361. Traditional Jacket Potatoes

Preparation time: 15 minutes
Cooking time: 25 minutes
Servings: 4
Ingredients:
4 potatoes, well washed
2 garlic cloves, minced
Salt and black pepper to taste
1 tsp rosemary
1 tsp butter
Directions:
Preheat your Air Fryer Oven to 360 F on Air Fry function. Prick the potatoes with a fork.
Put it into your Air fryer basket, then fit in the baking tray; cook for 25 minutes.
Cut the potatoes in half and top with butter and rosemary; season with salt and pepper. Serve immediately.
Nutrition:
Calories: 95
Carbs: 21g
Fat: 1g
Protein: 2g

362. Roasted Carrots

Preparation time: 15 minutes
Cooking time: 10 minutes
Servings: 4
Ingredients:
20 oz carrots, julienned
1 tbsp olive oil
1 tsp cumin seeds
2 tbsp fresh cilantro, chopped
Directions:
In a bowl, mix olive oil, carrots, and cumin seeds; stir to coat.
Place the carrots in a baking tray and cook in your on "Bake" function at 300 F for 10 minutes. Scatter fresh coriander over the carrots and serve.
Nutrition:
Calories: 89
Carbs: 10g
Fat: 6g
Protein: 1g

363. Garlicky Veggie Bake

Preparation time: 15 minutes
Cooking time: 15 minutes
Servings: 3
Ingredients:
3 turnips, sliced
1 large red onion, cut into rings
1 large zucchini, sliced
Salt and black pepper to taste
2 cloves garlic, crushed
1 bay leaf, cut into 6 pieces
1 tbsp olive oil
Directions:
Place the turnips, onion, and zucchini in a bowl. Toss with olive oil, salt, and pepper.
Preheat on Air Fry function to 380 F. Place the veggies into a baking pan.
Slip the bay leaves in the slices' different parts and tuck the garlic cloves between the slices—Cook for 15 minutes. Serve warm with as a side to a meat dish or salad.
Nutrition:
Calories: 140
Carbs: 26g
Fat: 4g
Protein: 1g

364. Sweet Baby Carrots

Preparation time: 15 minutes
Cooking time: 15 minutes
Servings: 4
Ingredients:
1-pound baby carrots
1 tsp dried dill
1 tbsp olive oil
1 tbsp honey
Salt and black pepper to taste
Directions:
Preheat your air fryer oven to 300 F on the "Air Fry" function.
In a bowl, mix oil, carrots, and honey; gently stir to coat—season with dill, pepper, and salt.
Place the carrots in the cooking basket and fit in the baking tray; cook for 15 minutes, shaking once. Serve.
Nutrition:
Calories: 35
Carbs: 9g
Fat: 0g
Protein: 0g

365. Colorful Vegetarian Delight

Preparation time: 15 minutes
Cooking time: 16 minutes
Servings: 2
Ingredients:
1 parsnip, sliced in a 2-inch thickness
1 cup chopped butternut squash
2 small red onions, cut into wedges
1 cup chopped celery
1 tbsp chopped fresh thyme
Salt and black pepper to taste
2 tsp olive oil
Directions:
Preheat on Air Fry function to 380 F.
In a bowl, add turnip, squash, red onions, celery, thyme, pepper, salt, and olive oil; mix well.
Add the veggies to the basket and fit in the baking tray; cook for 16 minutes, tossing once halfway through. Serve.
Nutrition:
Calories: 220
Carbs: 0g
Fat: 14g
Protein: 0g

366. Awesome Sweet Potato Fries

Preparation time: 15 minutes

Cooking time: 20 minutes
Servings: 4
Ingredients:
½ tsp salt
½ tsp garlic powder
½ tsp chili powder
¼ tsp cumin
3 tbsp olive oil
3 sweet potatoes, cut into thick strips
Directions:
In a bowl, mix salt, garlic powder, chili, and cumin, and olive oil.
Coat the strips well in this mixture and arrange them in the basket without overcrowding.
Fit in the baking tray and cook for 20 minutes at 380 F on Air Fry function or until crispy. Serve.
Nutrition:
Calories: 110
Carbs: 18g
Fat: 4g
Protein: 1g

367. Rosemary Butternut Squash Roast

Preparation time: 15 minutes
Cooking time: 20 minutes
Servings: 2
Ingredients:
1 butternut squash
1 tbsp dried rosemary
2 tbsp maple syrup
Salt to taste
Directions:
Slice the squash into wedges and season with salt. Preheat on Air Fry function to 350 F. Spray the wedges with cooking spray and sprinkle with rosemary.
Place the wedges in the basket without overlapping and fit in the baking tray. Cook within 20 minutes, flipping once halfway through. Serve with maple syrup and goat cheese.
Nutrition:
Calories: 136
Carbs: 25g
Fat: 5g
Protein: 2g

368. Cauliflower Rice with Tofu & Peas

Preparation time: 15 minutes
Cooking time: 22 minutes
Servings: 4
Ingredients:
Tofu:
½ block tofu, crumbled
½ cup diced onion
2 tbsp soy sauce
1 tsp turmeric
1 cup diced carrot
Cauliflower:
3 cups cauliflower rice
2 tbsp soy sauce
½ cup chopped broccoli
2 garlic cloves, minced
1 ½ tsp toasted sesame oil
1 tbsp minced ginger
½ cup frozen peas
1 tbsp rice vinegar
Directions:
Preheat on Air Fry function to 370 F. Combine all the tofu ingredients in a greased baking dish. Cook for 10 minutes.
Meanwhile, place all cauliflower ingredients in a large bowl and mix to combine.
Stir the cauliflower mixture in the tofu baking dish, return to the oven; cook for 12 minutes. Serve.
Nutrition:
Calories: 39
Carbs: 6g
Fat: 1g
Protein: 2g

369. Chickpea & Carrot Balls

Preparation time: 15 minutes
Cooking time: 18 minutes
Servings: 3
Ingredients:
2 tbsp olive oil
2 tbsp soy sauce
1 tbsp flax meal
2 cups cooked chickpeas
½ cup sweet onions
½ cup grated carrots
½ cup roasted cashews
Juice of 1 lemon
½ tsp turmeric
1 tsp cumin
1 tsp garlic powder
1 cup rolled oats
Directions:
Combine the olive oil, onions, and carrots into the Air Fryer baking pan and cook them on Air Fry function for 6 minutes at 350 F. Ground the oats and cashews in a food processor. Place in a large bowl. Mix in the chickpeas, lemon juice, and soy sauce.
Add onions and carrots to the bowl with chickpeas. Stir in the remaining ingredients; mix until fully incorporated. Make meatballs out of the mixture. Increase the temperature to 370 F and cook for 12 minutes.
Nutrition:
Calories: 189
Carbs: 7g
Fat: 17g
Protein: 2g

370. Yummy Chili Bean Burritos

Preparation time: 15 minutes
Cooking time: 5 minutes
Servings: 3
Ingredients:
6 tortillas
1 cup grated cheddar cheese
1 can (8 oz) beans
1 tsp Italian seasoning
Directions:
Preheat air fryer oven on Bake function to 350 F. Season the beans with the seasoning and divide them between the tortillas. Top with cheddar cheese. Roll

the burritos and arrange them on a lined baking dish. Cook for 5 minutes. Serve.

Nutrition:

Calories: 456
Carbs: 55g
Fat: 19g
Protein: 17g

371. Tasty Polenta Crisps

Preparation time: 15 minutes
Cooking time: 16 minutes
Servings: 4

Ingredients:

2 cups of milk
1 cup instant polenta
Salt and black pepper to taste
fresh thyme, chopped

Directions:

Fill a saucepan with milk and 2 cups of water and place over low heat. Bring it to a simmer.
Keep whisking as you pour in the polenta. Continue to whisk until polenta thickens and bubbles; season to taste. Add polenta to a lined with parchment paper baking tray and spread out.
Refrigerate for 45 minutes. Slice set polenta into batons and spray with olive oil.
Arrange polenta chips into the basket and fit in the baking tray; cook for 16 minutes at 380 F on Air Fry function, turning once halfway through. Serve.

Nutrition:

Calories: 80
Carbs: 16g
Fat: 1g
Protein: 2g

372. Crispy Pickles

Preparation Time: 10 minutes
Cooking Time: 6 minutes
Servings: 4

Ingredients:

16 dill pickles, sliced
1 egg, lightly beaten
1/2 cup almond flour
3 tbsp parmesan cheese, grated
1/2 cup pork rind, crushed

Directions:

Take three bowls. Mix pork rinds and cheese in the first bowl.
In a second bowl, add the egg.
In the last bowl, add the almond flour.
Coat each pickle slice with almond flour, then dip in egg and finally coat with pork and cheese mixture.
Spritz the air fryer basket with cooking spray. Place coated pickles in the air fryer basket.
Cook pickles for 6 minutes at 370 F. Serve and enjoy.

Nutrition:

Calories 245
Fat 17 g
Carbohydrates 4 g
Sugar 2 g
Protein 17 g
Cholesterol 41 mg

373. Asian Broccoli

Preparation Time: 10 minutes
Cooking Time: 20 minutes
Servings: 4

Ingredients:

1 lb. broccoli, cut into florets
1 tsp rice vinegar
2 tsp sriracha
2 tbsp soy sauce
1 tbsp garlic, minced
5 drops liquid stevia
1 1/2 tbsp sesame oil
Salt

Directions:

In a bowl, toss broccoli, garlic, oil, and salt.
Spread broccoli in the air fryer basket and cook for 15-20 minutes at 400 F.
Meanwhile, in a microwave-safe bowl, mix soy sauce, vinegar, liquid stevia, and sriracha and microwave for 10 seconds.
Transfer broccoli to a bowl and toss well with soy mixture to coat. Serve and enjoy.

Nutrition:

Calories 94
Fat 5.5 g
Carbohydrates 9.3 g
Sugar 2.1 g
Protein 3.8 g
Cholesterol 0 mg

374. Roasted Brussels Sprouts

Preparation Time: 10 minutes
Cooking Time: 8 minutes
Servings: 4

Ingredients:

1 lb. Brussels sprouts, cleaned and trimmed
1 tsp garlic powder
1 tsp dried parsley
2 tsp olive oil
1/2 tsp dried thyme
1/4 tsp salt

Directions:

Put all the fixing into the bowl and toss well. Pour Brussels sprout mixture into the air fryer basket.
Cook Brussels sprouts at 390 F for 8 minutes. Serve and enjoy.

Nutrition:

Calories 72
Fat 2.7 g
Carbohydrates 10.9 g
Sugar 2.6 g
Protein 4 g
Cholesterol 0 mg

375. Quick Creamy Spinach

Preparation Time: 10 minutes
Cooking Time: 15 minutes
Servings: 2

Ingredients:

10 oz frozen spinach, thawed
1/4 cup parmesan cheese, shredded
1/2 tsp ground nutmeg
1 tsp pepper
4 oz cream cheese, diced
2 tsp garlic, minced

1 small onion, chopped
1 tsp salt

Directions:

Spray 6-inch pan with cooking spray and set aside.
In a bowl, mix spinach, cream cheese, garlic, onion, nutmeg, pepper, and salt.
Pour spinach mixture into the prepared pan.
Put the dish in the air fryer basket and air fry at 350 F for 10 minutes.
Open the air fryer basket and sprinkle parmesan cheese on top of the spinach mixture and air fry at 400 F for 5 minutes more. Serve and enjoy.

Nutrition:

Calories 265
Fat 21.4 g
Carbohydrates 11.9 g
Sugar 2.4 g
Protein 10.2 g
Cholesterol 65 mg

376. Perfect Crispy Tofu

Preparation Time: 10 minutes
Cooking Time: 20 minutes
Servings: 4

Ingredients:

1 block firm tofu, cubes
1 tbsp arrowroot flour
2 tsp sesame oil
1 tsp vinegar
2 tbsp soy sauce

Directions:

In a bowl, toss tofu with oil, vinegar, and soy sauce and sit for 15 minutes.
Toss marinated tofu with arrowroot flour. Spray with the cooking spray the air fryer basket.
Add tofu in air fryer basket and cook for 20 minutes at 370 F, then shake it halfway through.
Serve and enjoy.

Nutrition:

Calories 42
Fat 0.5 g
Carbohydrates 1.3 g
Sugar 0.3g
Protein 12.4 g
Cholesterol 0 mg

377. Mushroom Bean Casserole

Preparation Time: 10 minutes
Cooking Time: 12 minutes
Servings: 6

Ingredients:

2 cups mushrooms, sliced
1 tsp onion powder
1/2 tsp ground sage
1/2 tbsp garlic powder
1 fresh lemon juice
1 1/2 lbs. green beans, trimmed
1/4 tsp pepper
1/2 tsp salt

Directions:

In a large mixing bowl, toss green beans, onion powder, sage, garlic powder, lemon juice, mushrooms, pepper, and salt.
Grease the air fryer basket using cooking spray—Transfer green bean mixture into the air fryer basket.
Cook for 10-12 minutes at 400 F. Shake after every 3 minutes. Serve and enjoy.

Nutrition:

Calories 45
Fat 0.2 g
Carbohydrates 9.8 g
Sugar 2.3g
Protein 3 g
Cholesterol 0 mg

378. Crisp & Tender Brussels Sprouts

Preparation Time: 10 minutes
Cooking Time: 10 minutes
Servings: 2

Ingredients:

2 cups Brussels sprouts, sliced
1 tbsp balsamic vinegar
1 tbsp olive oil
1/4 tsp sea salt

Directions:

Put all the fixings into a bowl and toss well. Grease the air fryer basket with a cooking spray.
Transfer Brussels sprouts mixture into the air fryer basket.
Cook Brussels sprouts at 400 F for 10 minutes. Shake when it's halfway through. Serve and enjoy.

Nutrition:

Calories 100
Fat 7.3 g
Carbohydrates 8.1 g
Sugar 1.9 g
Protein 3 g
Cholesterol 0 mg

379. Asian Green Beans

Preparation Time: 5 minutes
Cooking Time: 10 minutes
Servings: 2

Ingredients:

8 oz green beans, trimmed
1 tsp sesame oil
1 tbsp tamari

Directions:

Toss all the fixing into the large mixing bowl. Grease air fryer basket using a cooking spray.
Transfer green beans in the air fryer basket and cook at 400 F for 10 minutes. Toss halfway through.
Serve and enjoy.

Nutrition:

Calories 58
Fat 2 g
Carbohydrates 8 g
Sugar 3 g
Protein 3 g
Cholesterol 0 mg

380. Roasted Squash

Preparation Time: 10 minutes
Cooking Time: 35 minutes
Servings: 6

Ingredients:

4 cups butternut squash, diced

1/4 cup dried cranberries
3 garlic cloves, minced
1 tbsp soy sauce
1 tbsp balsamic vinegar
1 tbsp olive oil
8 oz mushrooms, quartered
1 cup green onions, sliced

Directions:

In a large mixing bowl, mix squash, mushrooms, and green onion and set aside.
In a small bowl, whisk oil, garlic, vinegar, and soy sauce.
Pour oil mixture over squash and toss to coat.
Spritz air fryer basket with cooking spray.
Add squash mixture into the air fryer basket and cook for 30-35 minutes at 400 F. Shake after every 5 minutes.
Toss with cranberries and serve hot.

Nutrition:

Calories 82
Fat 2.6 g
Carbohydrates 14.5 g
Sugar 3.3 g
Protein 2.7 g
Cholesterol 0 mg

381. Roasted Eggplant

Preparation Time: 10 minutes
Cooking Time: 12 minutes
Servings: 2

Ingredients:

1 eggplant, washed and cubed
1/2 tsp garlic powder
1/4 tsp marjoram
1/4 tsp oregano
1 tbsp olive oil

Directions:

Drizzle your air fryer basket with cooking spray. Put all the items into the mixing bowl and toss well.
Transfer eggplant mixture into the air fryer basket and cook at 390 F for 6 minutes.
Toss well and cook for 6 minutes more. Serve and enjoy.

Nutrition:

Calories 120
Fat 7.5 g
Carbohydrates 14.2 g
Sugar 7.1 g
Protein 2.4 g
Cholesterol 0 mg

382. Curried Eggplant Slices

Preparation Time: 10 minutes
Cooking Time: 10 minutes
Servings: 2

Ingredients:

1 large eggplant, thick slices
1 garlic clove, minced
1 tbsp olive oil
1/2 tsp curry powder
1/8 tsp turmeric
Salt

Directions:

Preheat the air fryer to 300 F.
Put all the items into the large mixing bowl and toss to coat—transfer eggplant slices into the air fryer basket.
Cook eggplant slices for 10 minutes or until lightly brown, then shake on halfway.
Serve and enjoy.

Nutrition:

Calories 122
Fat 7.5 g
Carbohydrates 14.4 g
Sugar 6.9 g
Protein 2.4 g
Cholesterol 0 mg

383. Healthy Green Beans

Preparation Time: 5 minutes
Cooking Time: 6 minutes
Servings: 4

Ingredients:

1 lb. green beans, trimmed
Pepper
Salt

Directions:

Drizzle the air fryer basket using cooking spray.
Preheat the air fryer to 400 F.
Add green beans in the air fryer basket and season with pepper and salt.
Cook green beans for 6 minutes. Turn halfway through. Serve and enjoy.

Nutrition:

Calories 35
Fat 0.1 g
Carbohydrates 8.1 g
Sugar 1.6 g
Protein 2.1 g
Cholesterol 0 mg

384. Healthy Air Fryer Mushrooms

Preparation Time: 10 minutes
Cooking Time: 12 minutes
Servings: 2

Ingredients:

8 oz mushrooms, sliced
1 tbsp parsley, chopped
1 tsp soy sauce
1/2 tsp garlic powder
1 tbsp olive oil
Pepper
Salt

Directions:

Put all the listed items into the mixing bowl and toss well.
Transfer mushrooms in the air fryer basket and cook at 380 F for 10-12 minutes. Halfway through it, shake.
Serve and enjoy.

Nutrition:

Calories 89
Fat 7.4 g
Carbohydrates 4.6 g
Sugar 2.2 g
Protein 3.9 g
Cholesterol 0 mg

385. Tasty Okra

Preparation Time: 10 minutes
Cooking Time: 12 minutes
Servings: 2
Ingredients:
1/2 lb. okra, ends trimmed and sliced
1 tsp olive oil
1/2 tsp mango powder
1/2 tsp chili powder
1/2 tsp ground coriander
1/2 tsp ground cumin
1/8 tsp pepper
1/4 tsp salt
Directions:
Warm the air fryer to 350 F. Add all ingredients into the large bowl and toss well.
Lightly spritz the air fryer basket with cooking spray.
Transfer okra mixture into the air fryer basket and cook for 10 minutes. Shake basket halfway through.
Toss okra well and cook for 2 minutes more. Serve and enjoy.
Nutrition:
Calories 70
Fat 2.8 g
Carbohydrates 9.1 g
Sugar 1.7 g
Protein 2.4 g
Cholesterol 0 mg

386. Cabbage Wedges

Preparation Time: 10 minutes
Cooking Time: 14 minutes
Servings: 6
Ingredients:
1 small cabbage head, cut into wedges
3 tbsp olive oil
1/4 tsp red chili flakes
1/2 tsp fennel seeds
1 tsp garlic powder
1 tsp onion powder
Pepper
Salt
Directions:
Grease the air fryer basket using cooking spray.
In a small bowl, mix garlic powder, red chili flakes, fennel seeds, onion powder, pepper, and salt.
Coat cabbage wedges with oil and rub with garlic powder mixture.
Place cabbage wedges into the air fryer basket and cook at 400 F for 8 minutes.
Turn cabbage wedges to another side and cook for 6 minutes more. Serve and enjoy.
Nutrition:
Calories 101
Fat 7.2 g
Carbohydrates 9.5 g
Sugar 5.1 g
Protein 2.1 g
Cholesterol 0 mg

387. Mexican Topped Avocados

Preparation time: 15 minutes
Cooking time: 4 minutes
Servings: 2
Ingredients:
1 cup seeded and diced tomatoes
1 tablespoon fresh lime juice
1 teaspoon lime zest
2 tablespoons chopped fresh cilantro
1 small jalapeño, seeded and minced
2 cloves garlic, peeled and minced
1 tablespoon peeled and diced red onion
½ teaspoon salt
2 large avocados, halved and pitted
4 tablespoons vegan Cheddar shreds
Directions:
Combine tomatoes, lime juice, lime zest, cilantro, jalapeño, garlic, onion, and salt in a medium bowl.
Cover and refrigerate until ready to use.
Warm the air fryer at 350°F for 3 minutes.
Place avocado halves, cut sides up, in an ungreased air fryer. Distribute cheese shreds to top of avocado halves. Cook 4 minutes.
Transfer avocados to a large serving plate, garnish with tomato mixture and serve.
Nutrition:
Calories: 172
Protein: 2g
Fiber: 6g
Fat: 14g
Sodium: 349mg
Carbohydrates: 12g
Sugar: 2g

388. Jackfruit "Fish" Fritters

Preparation time: 15 minutes
Cooking time: 20 minutes
Servings: 4
Ingredients:
1 can jackfruit, drained and chopped
1 flax egg
1 tablespoon Dijon mustard
1 tablespoon vegan mayonnaise
1 tablespoon prepared horseradish
2 tablespoons peeled and grated yellow onion
2 tablespoons chopped fresh parsley
2 tablespoons chopped nori
2 tablespoons almond flour
1 tablespoon Cajun seasoning
¼ teaspoon garlic powder
¼ teaspoon salt
2 lemon wedges
Directions:
Combine all fixings except lemon wedges in a medium bowl. Refrigerate covered 15 minutes.
Warm the air fryer at 350°F for 3 minutes. Cut a piece of parchment paper to fit the bottom of the air fryer basket.
Form chilled mixture into twelve balls, approximately 2 tablespoons each. Place six balls in an ungreased air fryer basket. Cook 10 minutes.
Transfer to a large plate and repeat cooking with remaining balls. Serve warm garnished with lemon wedges.
Nutrition:
Calories: 104
Protein: 1g
Fiber: 6g
Fat: 5g

Sodium: 413mg
Carbohydrates: 11g
Sugar: 4g

389. Vegetable-Stuffed Mushrooms

Preparation time: 15 minutes
Cooking time: 5 minutes
Servings: 2
Ingredients:
3 teaspoons olive oil, divided
12 whole white button mushroom caps
2 tablespoons diced white button mushroom stems
2 tablespoons small-diced yellow squash
1 teaspoon nutritional yeast
¼ teaspoon salt
2 tablespoons no-sugar-added tomato paste
1 tablespoon chopped fresh parsley
Directions:
Brush 1 teaspoon olive oil around the top ridge of mushroom caps.
Warm the air fryer at 350°F for 3 minutes.
In a medium bowl, combine mushroom stems, squash, nutritional yeast, salt, remaining olive oil, and tomato paste. Distribute and press mixture into tops of mushroom caps.
Place stuffed mushrooms in an ungreased air fryer basket. Cook 5 minutes.
Transfer mushrooms to a medium plate and garnish with parsley. Serve.
Nutrition:
Calories: 85
Protein: 2g
Fiber: 1g
Fat: 7g
Sodium: 305mg
Carbohydrates: 5g
Sugar: 3g

390. BBQ Jackfruit Lettuce Wraps with Coleslaw

Preparation time: 10 minutes
Cooking time: 10 minutes
Servings: 3
Ingredients:
1 cup prepackaged coleslaw mix
¼ cup vegan mayonnaise
2 teaspoons granular erythritol
½ teaspoon apple cider vinegar
¼ teaspoon salt
¼ teaspoon freshly ground black pepper
For Jackfruit Wraps:
1 can jackfruit in brine, diced
2/3 cup sugar-free BBQ sauce divided
6 large leaves iceberg lettuce
Directions:
Mix all the fixings in a medium bowl to make coleslaw. Refrigerate covered until ready to use.
To make Jackfruit Wraps: Preheat air fryer at 375°F for 3 minutes.
Toss 1/3 cup barbecue sauce with jackfruit in a medium bowl.
Place jackfruits in an air fryer basket lightly greased with olive oil and cook 5 minutes. Shake basket—Cook an additional 5 minutes.
Transfer jackfruits to a medium bowl. Add remaining sauce. Using two forks, pull apart jackfruit until it resembles pulled pork.
Serve jackfruit on lettuce leaves topped with coleslaw.
Nutrition:
Calories: 193
Protein: 1g
Fiber: 9g
Fat: 10g
Sodium: 895mg
Carbohydrates: 22g
Sugar: 25g

391. Greek Eggplant Rounds

Preparation time: 15 minutes
Cooking time: 10 minutes
Servings: 4
Ingredients:
2 teaspoons olive oil
1 long, narrow eggplant, sliced into rounds
½ teaspoon salt
½ cup no-sugar-added marinara sauce
½ cup feta cheese crumbles
8 kalamata olives, pitted and halved
2 tablespoons chopped fresh dill
Directions:
Warm air fryer at 350°F for 3 minutes.
Rub olive oil over both sides of eggplant circles.
Layout slices on a large plate and season evenly with salt. Top evenly with marinara sauce, feta crumbles, and olives.
Place half of the eggplant pizzas in an ungreased air fryer basket. Cook 5 minutes. Transfer back to the plate. Repeat cooking with remaining pizzas.
Garnish with chopped dill and serve warm.
Nutrition:
Calories: 82
Protein: 2g
Fiber: 2g
Fat: 5g
Sodium: 387mg
Carbohydrates: 7g
Sugar: 4g

392. Curried Tofu and Turmeric Cauli Rice

Preparation time: 5 minutes
Cooking time: 16 minutes
Servings: 4
Ingredients:
8 ounces extra-firm tofu, cubes
½ cup canned unsweetened coconut milk
2 teaspoons red curry paste
2 cloves garlic, peeled and minced
1 tablespoon avocado oil
1 tablespoon coconut oil
1 small head cauliflower, pulsed into rice
1 tablespoon turmeric powder
½ teaspoon salt
½ teaspoon freshly ground white pepper
4 lime wedges
¼ cup chopped fresh cilantro
Directions:

In a medium bowl, combine tofu, coconut milk, red curry paste, garlic, and avocado oil. Refrigerate covered 30 minutes.
Warm the air fryer at 350°F for 3 minutes.
Place tofu and marinade in an ungreased cake barrel, then put it in an air fryer basket and cook 5 minutes. Stir, then cook an additional 5 minutes.
While tofu is cooking, heat coconut oil in a medium skillet over medium-high heat for 30 seconds. Add rice cauliflower, turmeric powder, salt, and pepper. Stir-fry 6 minutes until cauliflower is tender to your preference.
Add cauliflower to four medium bowls. Top with tofu mixture and sauce. Garnish with lime wedges and cilantro. Serve warm.

Nutrition:
Calories: 177
Protein: 9g
Fiber: 4g
Fat: 12g
Sodium: 532mg
Carbohydrates: 12g
Sugar: 3g

393. Korean Ground "Beef" and Kimchi Bowls

Preparation time: 15 minutes
Cooking time: 8 minutes
Servings: 4

Ingredients:
2 cups beefless grounds
1 medium carrot, peeled and julienned
6 scallions, sliced, 2 tablespoons greens reserved for garnish
1 medium zucchini, diced
2 tablespoons coconut aminos
2 teaspoons sesame oil
1 teaspoon apple cider vinegar
2 teaspoons granular erythritol
1 tablespoon gochujang
¼ teaspoon salt
½ cup kimchi
2 teaspoons roasted sesame seeds

Directions:
Warm air fryer at 350°F for 3 minutes.
In a large bowl, combine beefless grounds, carrot, scallions, zucchini, coconut aminos, sesame oil, apple cider vinegar, erythritol, gochujang, and salt.
Place mixture in an ungreased cake barrel. Place the barrel in the air fryer basket and cook 6 minutes. Stir in kimchi—Cook an additional 2 minutes.
Transfer to two medium bowls and garnish with reserved scallion greens and roasted sesame seeds. Serve.

Nutrition:
Calories: 157
Protein: 15g
Fiber: 4g
Fat: 7g
Sodium: 762mg
Carbohydrates: 14g
Sugar: 6g

394. Caprese Hasselback Tomatoes

Preparation time: 15 minutes
Cooking time: 4 minutes
Servings: 3

Ingredients:
4 medium Roma tomatoes, bottoms removed to create flat surfaces
16 fresh basil leaves
1 (8-ounce) ball fresh mozzarella, sliced and then cut into 16 pieces
½ teaspoon salt
½ teaspoon freshly ground black pepper
1 tablespoon olive oil
2 teaspoons balsamic vinegar

Directions:
Preheat air fryer at 325°F for 3 minutes.
Make four even slices on each tomato, three-quarters of the way down. Stuff one basil leaf and a piece of mozzarella into each slice. Season with salt and pepper.
Place stuffed tomatoes in an ungreased air fryer basket. Cook 3 minutes. Transfer to a large serving plate.
Drizzle tomatoes with olive oil and balsamic vinegar and serve.

Nutrition:
Calories: 201
Protein: 12g
Fiber: 2g
Fat: 15g
Sodium: 522mg
Carbohydrates: 5g
Sugar: 4g

395. Stuffed Bell Peppers

Preparation time: 15 minutes
Cooking time: 22 minutes
Servings: 4

Ingredients:
2 medium bell peppers, the color of choice
4 teaspoons olive oil, divided
½ medium yellow onion, peeled and finely diced
¾ cup finely diced summer squash
¾ cup chopped baby Bella (cremini) mushrooms
½ cup canned fire-roasted diced tomatoes, including juice
¼ cup tomato sauce
2 teaspoons Italian seasoning
¼ teaspoon smoked paprika
½ teaspoon salt
¼ teaspoon freshly ground black pepper

Directions:
Slice the bell peppers in half, then seed them. Brush inside and tops of bell peppers with 2 teaspoons olive oil. Set aside.
In a medium skillet, heat remaining oil over medium-high heat 30 seconds. Add onion, squash, and mushrooms. Stir-fry 5 minutes until onions are tender.
Mix tomatoes, tomato sauce, Italian seasoning, smoked paprika, salt, and pepper in a medium bowl.
Warm the air fryer at 350°F for 3 minutes.
Evenly distribute mixture among the bell pepper halves.

Place two halves in the air fryer basket. Cook 8 minutes.
Transfer to a serving plate. Continue with remaining halves. Serve warm.
Nutrition:
Calories: 81
Protein: 2g
Fiber: 3g
Fat: 5g
Sodium: 409mg
Carbohydrates: 8g
Sugar: 5g

396. Creamy Pesto Spaghetti Squash

Preparation time: 15 minutes
Cooking time: 25 minutes
Servings: 4
Ingredients:
2 teaspoons olive oil
1 (1½-pound) spaghetti squash, halved and seeded
½ teaspoon salt, divided
½ cup pesto
½ cup ricotta cheese
2 tablespoons chopped fresh basil leaves
Directions:
Warm air fryer at 375°F for 3 minutes.
Rub olive oil over both halves of spaghetti squash. Season it with half of the salt. Place both halves, flat sides down, in an ungreased air fryer basket. Cook 25 minutes.
Transfer squash to a cutting board and let cool for 5 minutes until easy to handle. Once cooled, use a fork to gently pull the strands out of squash and place into a medium bowl.
Toss squash noodles with pesto, ricotta cheese, and remaining salt. Garnish with basil leaves. Serve warm.
Nutrition:
Calories: 243
Protein: 6g
Fiber: 3g
Fat: 20g
Sodium: 647mg
Carbohydrates: 12g
Sugar: 5g

397. Broccoli Casserole

Preparation time: 15 minutes
Cooking time: 14 minutes
Servings: 4
Ingredients:
4 cups steamed broccoli florets, chopped
¼ cup peeled diced yellow onion
½ cup diced white mushrooms
1 large egg
2 tablespoons sour cream
¼ cup mayonnaise
1 teaspoon salt
½ teaspoon freshly ground black pepper
1 cup coarsely crushed Cheddar cheese crisp
Directions:
In a large bowl, combine broccoli, onion, mushrooms, egg, sour cream, mayonnaise, salt, and pepper. Spoon mixture into a round cake barrel.
Warm the air fryer at 350°F for 3 minutes.
Cook casserole 14 minutes.
Remove barrels from the air fryer and let rest 10 minutes. Evenly distribute crushed Cheddar Cheese crisps over the top of the casserole and serve warm.
Nutrition:
Calories: 251
Protein: 10g
Fiber: 3g
Fat: 21g
Sodium: 896mg
Carbohydrates: 8g
Sugar: 2g

398. Vegan Dogs and Sauerkraut

Preparation time: 15 minutes
Cooking time: 5 minutes
Servings: 2
Ingredients:
4 vegan hot dogs
2 cups sauerkraut
2 tablespoons German mustard
Directions:
Preheat air fryer to 400°F for 3 minutes.
Add hot dogs to an ungreased air fryer basket. Cook 5 minutes.
Transfer hot dogs to a large plate and serve warm with sauerkraut and mustard.
Nutrition:
Calories: 137
Protein: 16g
Fiber: 6g
Fat: 2g
Sodium: 1,965mg
Carbohydrates: 16g
Sugar: 6g

399. Balsamic Artichokes

Preparation Time: 10 minutes
Cooking time: 7 minutes
Servings: 4
Ingredients:
4 big artichokes, trimmed
Salt and black pepper to the taste
2 tablespoons lemon juice
¼ cup extra virgin olive oil
2 teaspoons balsamic vinegar
1 teaspoon oregano, dried
2 garlic cloves, minced
Directions:
Spice artichokes with salt and pepper, rub them with half of the oil and half of the lemon juice, put them in your air fryer, and cook at 360 °F for 7 minutes.
Meanwhile, in a bowl, mix the rest of the lemon juice with vinegar, the remaining oil, salt, pepper, garlic, and oregano and stir very well.
Arrange artichokes on a platter, drizzle the balsamic vinaigrette over them and serve.
Nutrition:
Calories: 50
Carbs: 13g
Fat: 0g
Protein: 4g

400. Cheesy Artichokes

Preparation Time: 10 minutes
Cooking time: 6 minutes
Servings: 6
Ingredients:
14 ounces canned artichoke hearts
8 ounces cream cheese
16 ounces parmesan cheese, grated
10 ounces spinach
1/2 cup chicken stock
8 ounces mozzarella, shredded
1/2 cup sour cream
3 garlic cloves, minced
1/2 cup mayonnaise
1 teaspoon onion powder
Directions:
Mix the artichokes with stock, garlic, spinach, cream cheese, sour cream, onion powder, and mayo in a pan that fits your air fryer.
Toss, then introduce in your air fryer and cook at 350 °F for 6 minutes.
Add mozzarella and parmesan, stir well and serve.
Nutrition:
Calories: 110
Carbs: 12g
Fat: 6g
Protein: 5g

401. Artichokes and Special Sauce

Preparation Time: 10 minutes
Cooking time: 6 minutes
Servings: 2
Ingredients:
2 artichokes, trimmed
A drizzle of olive oil
2 garlic cloves, minced
1 tablespoon lemon juice
For the sauce:
¼ cup of coconut oil
¼ cup extra virgin olive oil
3 anchovy fillets
3 garlic cloves
Directions:
In a bowl, mix artichokes with oil, 2 garlic cloves, and lemon juice, toss well, transfer to your air fryer, cook at 350 °F for 6 minutes and divide among plates.
In your food processor, mix coconut oil with anchovy, 3 garlic cloves, and olive oil, blend very well, drizzle over artichokes and serve.
Nutrition:
Calories: 50
Carbs: 7g
Fat: 2g
Protein: 3g

402. Beet Salad and Parsley Dressing

Preparation Time: 10 minutes
Cooking time: 14 minutes
Servings: 4
Ingredients:
4 beets
2 tablespoons balsamic vinegar
A bunch of parsley, diced
Salt and black pepper to the taste
1 tablespoon extra-virgin olive oil
1 garlic clove, diced
2 tablespoons capers
Directions:
Put beets in your air fryer and cook them at 360 °F for 14minutes.
Meanwhile, in a bowl, mix parsley with garlic, salt, pepper, olive oil, and capers and stir very well.
Transfer beets to a cutting board, leave them to cool down, peel them, slice, and put them in a salad bowl.
Add vinegar, drizzle the parsley dressing all over and serve.
Nutrition:
Calories: 30
Carbs: 1g
Fat: 3g
Protein: 0g

403. Beets and Blue Cheese Salad

Preparation Time: 10 minutes
Cooking time: 14 minutes
Servings: 6
Ingredients:
6 beets, peeled and quartered
Salt and black pepper to the taste
¼ cup blue cheese, crumbled
1 tablespoon olive oil
Directions:
Put beets in your air fryer, cook them at 350 °F for 14 minutes, and transfer them to a bowl.
Add blue cheese, salt, pepper, and oil, toss and serve.
Nutrition:
Calories: 370
Carbs: 34g
Fat: 23g
Protein: 12g

404. Beet, Tomato, and Goat Cheese Mix

Preparation Time: 30 minutes
Cooking time: 14 minutes
Servings: 8
Ingredients:
8 small beets, trimmed, peeled, and halved
1 red onion, sliced
4 ounces goat cheese, crumbled
1 tablespoon balsamic vinegar
Salt and black pepper to the taste
2 tablespoons sugar
1-pint mixed cherry tomatoes halved
2 ounces pecans
2 tablespoons olive oil
Directions:
Put beets in your air fryer, spice them with salt and pepper, cook at 350 °F for 14 minutes and transfer to a salad bowl.
Add onion, cherry tomatoes, and pecans and toss.
In another bowl, mix vinegar with sugar and oil, whisk well until sugar dissolves, and add to salad.
Also, add goat cheese, toss and serve.
Nutrition:
Calories: 267
Carbs: 19g
Fat: 20g
Protein: 7g

405. Broccoli Salad

Preparation Time: 10 minutes
Cooking time: 8 minutes4
Servings:
Ingredients:
1 broccoli head, florets separated
1 tablespoon peanut oil
6 garlic cloves, minced
1 tablespoon Chinese rice wine vinegar
Salt and black pepper to the taste
Directions:
In a bowl, mix broccoli with salt, pepper, and half of the oil, toss, transfer to your air fryer and cook at 350 °F for 8 minutes, shaking the fryer halfway.
Transfer broccoli to a salad bowl, add the rest of the peanut oil, garlic, and rice vinegar, toss well, and serve.
Nutrition:
Calories: 160
Carbs: 15g
Fat: 10g
Protein: 4g

406. Brussels Sprouts And Tomatoes Mix

Preparation Time: 5 minutes
Cooking time: 10 minutes
Servings: 4
Ingredients:
1-pound Brussels sprouts, trimmed
Salt and black pepper to the taste
6 cherry tomatoes, halved
¼ cup green onions, diced
1 tablespoon olive oil
Directions:
Spice Brussels sprouts with salt and pepper, put them in your air fryer, and cook at 350 °F for 10 minutes.
Transfer them to a bowl, add salt, pepper, cherry tomatoes, green onions, and olive oil, toss well and serve.
Nutrition:
Calories: 60
Carbs: 2g
Fat: 0g
Protein: 1g

407. Brussels Sprouts And Butter Sauce

Preparation Time: 4 minutes
Cooking time: 10 minutes
Servings: 4
Ingredients:
1-pound Brussels sprouts, trimmed
Salt and black pepper to the taste
1/2 cup bacon, cooked and diced
1 tablespoon mustard
1 tablespoon butter
2 tablespoons dill, finely diced
Directions:
Put Brussels sprouts in your air fryer and cook them at 350 degrees F for 10 minutes.
Warm a pan with the butter over medium-high heat, add bacon, mustard, and dill and whisk well.
Divide Brussels sprouts on plates, drizzle butter sauce all over, and serve.
Nutrition:
Calories: 70
Carbs: 9g
Fat: 2g
Protein: 3g

408. Cheesy Brussels Sprouts

Preparation Time: 10 minutes
Cooking time: 8 minutes
Servings: 4
Ingredients:
1-pound Brussels sprouts washed
Juice of 1 lemon
Salt and black pepper to the taste
2 tablespoons butter
3 tablespoons parmesan, grated
Directions:
Put Brussels sprouts in your air fryer, cook them at 350 °F for 8 minutes and transfer them to a bowl.
Warm a pan with the butter over medium heat, add lemon juice, salt, and pepper, whisk well and add to Brussels sprouts.
Add parmesan, toss until parmesan melts and serve.
Nutrition:
Calories: 240
Carbs: 26g
Fat: 9g
Protein: 12g

409. Spicy Cabbage

Preparation Time: 10 minutes
Cooking time: 8 minutes
Servings: 4
Ingredients:
1 cabbage, cut into 8 wedges
1 tablespoon sesame seed oil
1 carrot, grated
¼ cup apple cider vinegar
¼ cups apple juice
1/2 teaspoon cayenne pepper
1 teaspoon red pepper flakes, crushed
Directions:
Mix the cabbage with oil, carrot, vinegar, apple juice, cayenne, and pepper flakes in a pan that fits your air fryer, introduce in the preheated air fryer, and cook 350 °F for 8 minutes.
Divide cabbage mix among plates and serve.
Nutrition:
Calories: 151
Carbs: 6g
Fat: 8g
Protein: 13g

410. Sweet Baby Carrots Dish

Preparation Time: 10 minutes
Cooking time: 10 minutes
Servings: 4
Ingredients:
2 cups baby carrots
A pinch of salt and black pepper
1 tablespoon brown sugar
1/2 tablespoon butter, melted

Directions:

In a dish that fits your air fryer, mix baby carrots with butter, salt, pepper, sugar, toss, introduce in your air fryer and cook at 350 °F for 10 minutes.

Divide among plates and serve.

Nutrition:

Calories: 35
Carbs: 9g
Fat: 0g
Protein: 0g

411. Herbed Eggplant and Zucchini Mix

Preparation Time: 10 minutes
Cooking time: 8 minutes
Servings: 4

Ingredients:

1 eggplant, roughly cubed
3 zucchinis, roughly cubed
2 tablespoons lemon juice
Salt and black pepper to the taste
1 teaspoon thyme, dried
1 teaspoon oregano, dried
3 tablespoons olive oil

Directions:

Put eggplant in a dish that fits your air fryer, add zucchinis, lemon juice, salt, pepper, thyme, oregano, and olive oil, toss, introduce in your air fryer and cook at 360 °F for 8 minutes.

Divide among plates and serve right away.

Nutrition:

Calories: 190
Carbs: 15g
Fat: 11g
Protein: 11g

412. Flavored Fennel

Preparation Time: 10 minutes
Cooking time: 8 minutes
Servings: 4

Ingredients:

2 fennel bulbs, cut into quarters
3 tablespoons olive oil
Salt and black pepper to the taste
1 garlic clove, minced
1 red chili pepper, diced
¾ cup veggie stock
Juice from 1/2 lemon
¼ cup white wine
¼ cup parmesan, grated

Directions:

Heat a pan that fits your air fryer with the oil over medium-high heat, add garlic and chili pepper, stir and cook for 2 minutes.

Add fennel, salt, pepper, stock, wine, lemon juice, and parmesan, toss to coat, introduce in your air fryer and cook at 350 °F for 6 minutes.

Divide among plates and serve right away.

Nutrition:

Calories: 12
Carbs: 2g
Fat: 0g
Protein: 1g

413. Crispy Potatoes and Parsley

Preparation Time: 10 minutes
Cooking time: 10 minutes
Servings: 4

Ingredients:

1-pound gold potatoes, cut into wedges
Salt and black pepper to the taste
2 tablespoons olive
Juice from ½ lemon
¼ cup parsley leaves, chopped

Directions:

Rub potatoes with salt, pepper, lemon juice, and olive oil, put them in your air fryer, and cook at 350°F for 10 minutes.

Divide among plates, sprinkle parsley on top, and serve.

Nutrition:

Calories: 201
Carbs: 35g
Fat: 5g
Protein: 4g

Chapter 9. Dehydrated

414. Dehydrated Pineapple Slices

Preparation Time: 10 minutes
Cooking Time: 14 hours
Servings: 12
Ingredients:
1 small pineapple, trim, peel, and cut into 1/8-inch thick slices
Directions:
Arrange pineapple slices on the dehydrate basket in a single layer.
Set temperature 125 F, then dehydrate pineapple slices for 14 hours.
Nutrition:
Calories 376
Fat 0.9 g
Carbohydrates 99.2 g
Sugar 74.5 g
Protein 4.1 g
Cholesterol 0 mg

415. Dehydrated Mango Slices

Preparation Time: 10 minutes
Cooking Time: 12 hours
Servings: 4
Ingredients:
2 mangoes, peel, and cut into 1/4-inch thick slices
Directions:
Arrange mango slices on the dehydrate basket in a single layer.
Set temperature 135 F. Dehydrate mango slices for 12 hours.
Nutrition:
Calories 101
Fat 0.6 g
Carbohydrates 25.2 g
Sugar 23 g
Protein 1.4 g
Cholesterol 0 mg

416. Dehydrated Green Apple Slices

Preparation Time: 10 minutes
Cooking Time: 8 hours
Servings: 4
Ingredients:
2 green apples, 1/8-inch thick slices
1 tsp ground cinnamon
Directions:
Arrange green apple slices on the dehydrate basket in a single layer. Sprinkle cinnamon on top of apple slices.
Set temperature 145 F. Dehydrate green apple slices for 8 hours.
Nutrition:
Calories 59
Fat 0.2 g
Carbohydrates 15.9 g
Sugar 11.6 g
Protein 0.3 g
Cholesterol 0 mg

417. Dehydrated Raspberries

Preparation Time: 10 minutes
Cooking Time: 12 hours
Servings: 4
Ingredients:
2 cups fresh raspberries, wash and pat dry with a paper towel
Directions:
Arrange raspberries on the dehydrate basket in a single layer.
Set temperature 135 F, then dehydrate raspberries for 12 hours.
Nutrition:
Calories 32
Fat 0.4 g
Carbohydrates 7.3 g
Sugar 2.7 g
Protein 0.7 g
Cholesterol 0 mg

418. Candied Pecans

Preparation Time: 10 minutes
Cooking Time: 12 hours
Servings: 4
Ingredients:
1 cup pecan halves, soaked in water overnight
6 tbsp maple syrup
Pinch of cinnamon
Directions:
In a bowl, toss pecan with maple syrup and cinnamon and arrange on the dehydrate basket.
Dehydrate pecans for 12 hours at temperature 125 F.
Nutrition:
Calories 103
Fat 2.6 g
Carbohydrates 20.7 g
Sugar 18 g
Protein 0.4 g
Cholesterol 0 mg

419. Dehydrated Avocado Slices

Preparation Time: 10 minutes
Cooking Time: 10 hours
Servings: 4
Ingredients:
3 avocados, halved, pitted, and cut into slices
1/4 tsp red chili powder
Directions:
Arrange avocado slices on the dehydrate basket in a single layer. Sprinkle chili powder over avocado slices.
Dehydrate avocado slices at temperature 160 F for 10 hours.
Nutrition:
Calories 308
Fat 29.4 g
Carbohydrates 13.1 g
Sugar 0.8 g
Protein 2.9 g
Cholesterol 0 mg

420. Dehydrated Eggplant Slices

Preparation Time: 10 minutes
Cooking Time: 4 hours

Servings: 4
Ingredients:
1 eggplant, 1/4-inch thick slices
Directions:
Arrange eggplant slices on the dehydrate basket in a single layer.
Dehydrate eggplant slices temperature 145 F for 4 hours.
Nutrition:
Calories 29
Fat 0.2 g
Carbohydrates 6.7 g
Sugar 3.4 g
Protein 1.1 g
Cholesterol 0 mg

421. Dehydrated Zucchini Chips

Preparation Time: 10 minutes
Cooking Time: 8 hours
Servings: 4
Ingredients:
2 zucchinis, cut into 1/4-inch thick slices
1 tsp olive oil
Pepper
Salt
Directions:
Toss zucchini slices with oil, pepper, and salt and arrange the dehydrate basket in a single layer.
Dehydrate zucchini slices temperature 135 F for 8 hours.
Nutrition:
Calories 26
Fat 1.4 g
Carbohydrates 3.3 g
Sugar 1.7 g
Protein 1.2 g
Cholesterol 0 mg

422. Dehydrated Strawberry Slices

Preparation Time: 10 minutes
Cooking Time: 12 hours
Servings: 4
Ingredients:
1 cup strawberries, cut into 1/8-inch thick slices
Directions:
Arrange strawberry slices on the dehydrate basket in a single layer.
Dehydrate strawberry slices at temperature 130 F for 12 hours.
Nutrition:
Calories 12
Fat 0.1 g
Carbohydrates 2.8 g
Sugar 1.8 g
Protein 0.2 g
Cholesterol 0 mg

423. Dehydrated Sweet Potato Slices

Preparation Time: 10 minutes
Cooking Time: 12 hours
Servings: 4
Ingredients:
1 large sweet potato, sliced thinly
Directions:
Arrange sweet potato slices on the dehydrate basket in a single layer.
Dehydrate sweet potato slices at temperature 125 F for 12 hours.
Nutrition:
Calories 41
Fat 0.1 g
Carbohydrates 9.3 g
Sugar 2.9 g
Protein 0.9 g
Cholesterol 0 mg

424. Dehydrated Cucumber Chips

Preparation Time: 10 minutes
Cooking Time: 12 hours
Servings: 3
Ingredients:
1 cucumber, sliced
Pepper
Salt
Directions:
Arrange cucumber slices on the dehydrate basket in a single layer. Season with pepper and salt.
Dehydrate cucumber slices at temperature 135 F for 12 hours.
Nutrition:
Calories 15
Fat 0.1 g
Carbohydrates 3.7 g
Sugar 1.7 g
Protein 0.7 g
Cholesterol 0 mg

425. Dehydrated Broccoli Florets

Preparation Time: 10 minutes
Cooking Time: 12 hours
Servings: 6
Ingredients:
1 lb. broccoli florets
Pepper
Salt
Directions:
Arrange broccoli florets on the dehydrate basket in a single layer, then put pepper and salt.
Dehydrate broccoli florets at temperature 115 F for 12 hours.
Nutrition:
Calories 26
Fat 0.3 g
Carbohydrates 5 g
Sugar 1.3 g
Protein 2.1 g
Cholesterol 0 mg

426. Dehydrated Beet Slices

Preparation Time: 10 minutes
Cooking Time: 10 hours
Servings: 2
Ingredients:
1 beet, sliced thinly
Salt
Directions:
Arrange beet slices on the dehydrate basket in a single layer. Season with salt.

Dehydrate beet slices at temperature 135 F for 10 hours.

Nutrition:

Calories 22
Fat 0.1 g
Carbohydrates 5 g
Sugar 4 g
Protein 0.8 g
Cholesterol 0 mg

427. Dehydrated Tomato Slices

Preparation Time: 10 minutes
Cooking Time: 12 hours
Servings: 4

Ingredients:

4 tomatoes, sliced thinly
Pepper
Salt

Directions:

Arrange tomato slices on the dehydrate basket in a single layer. Season with pepper and salt.
Dehydrate tomato slices at temperature 135 F for 12 hours.

Nutrition:

Calories 22
Fat 0.3 g
Carbohydrates 4.8 g
Sugar 3.2 g
Protein 1.1 g
Cholesterol 0 mg

428. Dehydrated Green Beans

Preparation Time: 10 minutes
Cooking Time: 12 hours
Servings: 4

Ingredients:

1 lb. green beans
Salt

Directions:

Arrange green beans on the dehydrate basket in a single layer. Season with salt.
Dehydrate green beans at temperature 125 F for 12 hours.

Nutrition:

Calories 35
Fat 0.1 g
Carbohydrates 8.1 g
Sugar 1.6 g
Protein 2.1 g
Cholesterol 0 mg

Chapter 10. Desserts

429. Cinnamon Toast

Preparation time: 10 minutes
Cooking time: 5 minutes
Servings: 6

Ingredients:

2 tsp. pepper
1½ tsp. vanilla extract
1½ tsp. cinnamon
Sweetener of choice
1 cup of coconut oil
12 slices whole-wheat bread

Directions:

Melt coconut oil and mix with sweetener until dissolved. Mix in remaining ingredients minus bread till incorporated.
Spread mixture onto bread, covering all areas. Pour the coated pieces of bread into the oven rack.
Place the rack on the middle shelf of the Air Fryer Oven. Select TOAST—set temperature to 400°F and the time to 5 minutes.
Cut diagonally, and enjoy!

Nutrition:

Calories 124
Fat 2 g
Carbs 4 g
Protein 0 g

430. Chocolate Mug Cake

Preparation time: 7 minutes
Cooking time: 13 minutes
Servings: 6

Ingredients:

½ cup of cocoa powder
½ cup stevia powder
1 cup coconut cream
1 package cream cheese, room temperature
1 tbsp. vanilla extract
1 tbsp. butter

Directions:

Preheat the Air Fryer Oven within 5 minutes at 350°F.
Mix all the listed ingredients using a hand mixer until fluffy in a mixing bowl.
Pour into greased mugs. Place the mugs in the fryer basket.
Bake for 13 minutes at 350°F.
Serve when cool.

Nutrition:

Calories 744
Fat 69.7 g
Carbs 4 g
Protein 13.9 g.

431. Fried Peaches

Preparation time: 2 hours & 15 minutes
Cooking time: 15 minutes
Servings: 4

Ingredients:

4 ripe peaches
1½ cup flour
Salt, to taste
2 egg yolks
¾ cup of water
1½ tbsp. olive oil
2 tbsp. brandy
4 egg whites
Cinnamon/sugar mix

Directions:

Mix flour, egg yolks, and salt in a mixing bowl.
Slowly mix in ¾ cup water, then add brandy.
Set the mixture aside for 2 hours and meanwhile cut an X at the bottom of each peach.
Bring a large pot of water to a boil. Add peaches to boiling water for about a minute, then transfer to a large bowl of cold water. The peels should fall off the peach.
Beat the egg whites and mix into the batter.
Dip each peach in the mix to coat. Lightly grease the oven rack with olive oil.
Pour the coated peach into the oven rack. Place the rack on the middle shelf of the Air Fryer Oven.
Set temperature to 360°F, and set time to 10 minutes.
Prepare a plate with cinnamon/sugar mix, roll peaches in the mix and serve.

Nutrition:

Calories 306
Fat 3 g
Fiber 2.7 g
Protein 10 g

432. Apple Dumplings

Preparation time: 7 minutes
Cooking time: 25 minutes
Servings: 4

Ingredients:

2 tbsp. melted coconut oil
2 puff pastry sheets
1 tbsp. brown sugar
2 tbsp. raisins
2 small apples, wedges
Cooking spray

Directions:

Preheat your Air Fryer Oven to 356°F. Grease the baking pan, then set aside.
Mix the apple wedges with raisins and sugar in a bowl.
Place a bit of apple mixture into puff pastry sheets and brush sides with melted coconut oil. Fold over the apple mixture and seal.
Pour in the baking pan. Place into the air fryer.
Bake for 25 minutes, turning halfway through. Serve warm.

Nutrition:

Calories 367
Fat 7 g
Carbs 5 g
Protein 2 g

433. Apple Pie

Preparation time: 5 minutes
Cooking time: 30 minutes
Servings: 4

Ingredients:

½ tsp. vanilla extract
1 beaten egg

1 large apple, chopped
1 Pillsbury pie crust
1 tbsp. butter, sliced
1 tbsp. ground cinnamon
1 tbsp. raw sugar
2 tbsp. sugar
2 tsp. lemon juice
Cooking spray

Directions:

Lightly grease baking pan of Air Fryer Oven using cooking spray.
Put the pie crust on the pan up to the sides.
In a bowl, mix vanilla, lemon juice, raw sugar, cinnamon, and apples and pour on top of the pie crust.
Top the apples with butter slices, then cover it with the other pie crust.
Put the beaten egg on top of the crust and sprinkle sugar.
Bake for 30 minutes at 350°F. Serve and enjoy.

Nutrition:

Calories 372
Fat 19 g
Carbs 5 g
Protein 4.2 g

434. Air Fryer Chocolate Cake

Preparation time: 6 minutes
Cooking time: 35 minutes
Servings: 9

Ingredients:

½ cup hot water
1 tsp. vanilla extract
¼ cup olive oil
½ cup almond milk
1 egg
½ tsp. salt
¾ tsp. baking soda
¾ tsp. baking powder
½ cup unsweetened cocoa powder
2 cups almond flour
1 cup brown sugar

Directions:

Preheat your Air Fryer Oven to 356°F.
Mix all the dry items (brown sugar, flour, cocoa powder, baking powder, baking soda, and salt) in a large bowl.
Add vanilla extract, olive oil, milk, and egg in the dry mixture. Stir well until evenly mixed.
Add hot water last. Stir until the batter becomes thin.
Put the cake batter into a pan that fits into the fryer.
Bake for 35 minutes or if a toothpick inserted in the middle comes out clean.
When done, let stand for about 10 minutes before removing the cake from the pan.
Serve cool.

Nutrition:

Calories 378
Fat 9 g
Carbs 5 g
Protein 4 g.

435. Chocolate Soufflé

Preparation time: 7 minutes
Cooking time: 12 minutes
Servings: 2

Ingredients:

2 tbsp. almond flour
½ tsp. vanilla
3 tbsp. sweetener
2 separated eggs
¼ cup melted coconut oil
3 oz. of semi-sweet chocolate, chopped

Directions:

Preheat the Air Fryer Oven to 330°F.
Brush coconut oil and sweetener onto ramekins.
Melt coconut oil and chocolate.
Beat egg yolks well, adding vanilla and sweetener.
Stir in flour and ensure there are no lumps.
Whisk egg whites till they reach peak state and fold them into chocolate mixture. Mix until well blended.
Pour batter into ramekins and place into the Air Fryer Oven.
Then bake for 12 minutes or if a toothpick inserted in the middle comes out clean.
Serve with powdered sugar dusted on top.

Nutrition:

Calories 238
Fat 6 g
Carbs 4 g
Protein 1 g.

436. Saucy Fried Bananas

Preparation time: 7 minutes
Cooking time: 10 minutes
Servings: 2

Ingredients:

1 large egg
¼ cup cornstarch
¼ cup plain bread crumbs
3 bananas, halved crosswise
Cooking oil
Chocolate sauce

Directions:

Preheat your Air Fryer Oven to 350°F.
Whisk the egg in a small bowl.
Put the cornstarch in another bowl.
Put the bread crumbs in a different bowl.
Dip the bananas in the cornstarch, then the egg, and then the bread crumbs.
Spray the basket with cooking oil. Place the bananas in the basket and spray them with cooking oil.
Select AIR FRY. Cook for 5 minutes.
Turn over the bananas then cook again within 2 minutes.
Put the chocolate sauce over the bananas, then serve.

Nutrition:

Calories 203
Fat 6 g
Fiber 3 g
Protein 3 g.

437. Crusty Apple Hand Pies

Preparation time: 7 minutes
Cooking time: 8 minutes
Servings: 6

Ingredients:

15 oz. no-sugar-added apple pie filling

1 store-bought crust

Directions:

Layout pie crust and slice into equal-sized squares.
Place 2 tbsp filling into each square and seal the crust with a fork. Pour into the oven rack.
Place the rack on the middle shelf of the Air Fryer Oven.
Set temperature to 390°F, and bake within 8 minutes until golden in color. Serve hot.

Nutrition:

Calories 278
Fat 10 g
Carbs 4 g
Protein 5 g

438. Blueberry Lemon Muffins

Preparation time: 7 minutes
Cooking time: 8 minutes
Servings: 12

Ingredients:

1 tsp. vanilla extract
Juice and zest of 1 lemon
2 eggs
1 cup blueberries
½ cup cream
¼ cup avocado oil
½ cup monk fruit
2½ cup almond flour

Directions:

Preheat the oven to 320°F. Grease the muffin tin with avocado oil and set aside.
Mix monk fruit and flour in a bowl.
In another bowl, whisk vanilla extract, eggs, lemon juice, lemon zest, and cream.
Add mixtures and blend well. Carefully stir in the blueberries.
Spoon batter into muffin tin. Place in the Air Fryer Oven.
Bake within 8 minutes at 320°F, checking at 6 minutes to ensure you don't over bake them.
Cool completely before serving.

Nutrition:

Calories 317
Fat 11 g
Carbs 5 g
Protein 3 g.

439. Cream Cheese Wontons

Preparation time: 5 minutes
Cooking time: 5 minutes
Servings: 16

Ingredients:

1 egg, mixed with a bit of water
Wonton wrappers
½ cup powdered erythritol
8 oz. softened cream cheese
Olive oil cooking spray

Directions:

Mix sweetener and cream cheese.
Layout the four wonton wrappers at a time, then cover with a dish towel to prevent drying out.
Place ½ tsp. of cream cheese mixture into each wrapper.
Lightly brush the edges of wonton wrappers with egg mixture and fold diagonally to form a triangle.
Seal edges well and repeats the same with the remaining ingredients.
Place filled wontons onto the oven pan and then into the Air Fryer Oven.
Bake for 5 minutes at 400°F, shaking halfway through cooking. Serve hot.

Nutrition:

Calories 303
Fat 3 g
Carbs 4 g
Protein 0.5 g

440. Air Fryer Cinnamon Rolls

Preparation time: 2 hours & 11 minutes
Cooking time: 5 minutes
Servings: 8

Ingredients:

1½ tbsp. cinnamon
¾ cup brown sugar
¼ cup melted coconut oil
1 lb. frozen bread dough, thawed
Glaze:
½ tsp. vanilla
1¼ cups powdered erythritol
2 tbsp. softened ghee
3 oz. softened cream cheese

Directions:

Layout bread dough and roll out into a rectangle.
Brush melted ghee over the dough and leave a 1-inch border along the edges.
Mix cinnamon, brown sugar, coconut oil, and sweetener and then sprinkle over dough.
Roll dough tightly and slice into 8 pieces. Let sit for 2 hours to rise.
To make the glaze, simply mix the glaze ingredients till smooth.
Once rolls rise, place into the air fryer—Bake for 5 minutes at 350°F.
Serve rolls drizzled in cream cheese glaze. Enjoy!

Nutrition:

Calories 390
Fat 8 g
Carbs 7 g
Protein 1 g.

441. Cinnamon Fried Bananas

Preparation time: 7 minutes
Cooking time: 10 minutes
Servings: 3

Ingredients:

1 cup panko bread crumbs
3 tbsp. cinnamon
½ cup almond flour
3 egg whites
8 ripe bananas
3 tbsp. coconut oil

Directions:

Heat coconut oil and add bread crumbs, then mix around 3 minutes until golden and pour into a bowl.
In another bowl, pour in the egg whites. Add almond flour in a third dish.

Peel and cut bananas in half. Roll the half of each banana into flour, egg whites, and then crumb mixture. Sprinkle cinnamon on top.
Arrange the coated bananas on the oven pan. Place into the Air Fryer Oven.
Bake for 10 minutes at 280°F until crispy and brown.
Cool for 5 minutes before serving.
Nutrition:
Calories 219
Fat 10 g
Carbs 5 g
Protein 3 g

442. Banana Split

Preparation Time: 15 minutes
Cooking Time: 14 minutes
Servings: 8
Ingredients:
3 tablespoons coconut oil
1 cup panko breadcrumbs
½ cup of corn flour
2 eggs
4 bananas, peeled and halved lengthwise
3 tablespoons sugar
¼ teaspoon ground cinnamon
2 tablespoons walnuts, chopped
Directions:
Dissolve the coconut oil over medium heat in a medium skillet and cook breadcrumbs for about 3-4 minutes or until golden browned and crumbled, stirring continuously.
Transfer the breadcrumbs into a shallow bowl and set aside to cool.
In a second bowl, place the corn flour.
In a third bowl, whisk the eggs.
Coat the banana slices with flour, dip into eggs, and, finally, coat evenly with the breadcrumbs.
Mix the sugar plus cinnamon in a small bowl.
Air Fry within 10 minutes at 280 degrees F.
Arrange the banana slices in "Air Fry Basket" and sprinkle with cinnamon sugar.
Transfer the banana slices onto plates to cool slightly.
Sprinkle with chopped walnuts and serve.
Nutrition:
Calories 216
Fat 8.8g
Cholesterol 41 mg
Sodium 16 mg
Total Carbs 26 g
Fiber 2.3 g
Sugar 11.9 g
Protein 3.4 g

443. Crispy Banana Slices

Preparation Time: 15 minutes
Cooking Time: 15 minutes
Servings: 8
Ingredients:
4 medium ripe bananas, peeled
1/3 cup rice flour, divided
2 tablespoons all-purpose flour
2 tablespoons corn flour
2 tablespoons desiccated coconut
½ teaspoon baking powder
½ teaspoon ground cardamom
Pinch of salt
Water, as required
¼ cup sesame seeds
Directions:
Mix 2 tablespoons of rice flour, all-purpose flour, corn flour, coconut, baking powder, cardamom, and salt in a shallow bowl.
Gradually, add the water and mix until a thick and smooth mixture forms.
In a second bowl, place the remaining rice flour.
In a third bowl, add the sesame seeds.
Cut each banana into half and then cut each half in 2 pieces lengthwise.
Dip the banana slices into the coconut mixture and then coat with the remaining rice flour, followed by the sesame seeds.
Air Fry within 15 minutes at 390 degrees F.
Arrange the banana slices in "Air Fry Basket" and insert it in the oven.
Transfer the banana slices onto plates to cool slightly before serving.
Nutrition:
Calories 121
Fat 3 g
Cholesterol 0 mg
Sodium 21 mg
Total Carbs 23.1 g
Fiber 2.6 g
Sugar 7.3 g
Protein 2.2 g

444. Pineapple Bites

Preparation Time: 10 minutes
Cooking Time: 10 minutes
Servings: 4
Ingredients:
For Pineapple Sticks:
½ of pineapple
¼ cup desiccated coconut
For Yogurt Dip:
1 tablespoon fresh mint leaves, minced
1 cup vanilla yogurt
Directions:
Cut the pineapple into long 1-2-inch-thick sticks.
In a shallow dish, place the coconut.
Coat the pineapple sticks with coconut evenly.
Set on Air Fry, then the cooking time within 10 minutes at 390 degrees F.
Arrange the pineapple sticks in lightly greased "Air Fry Basket" and insert it in the oven.
Meanwhile, for a dip in a bowl, mix mint and yogurt.
Serve pineapple sticks with yogurt dip.
Nutrition:
Calories 124
Fat 2.6 g
Cholesterol 4 mg
Sodium 46 mg
Total Carbs 21.6 g
Fiber 2.3 g
Sugar 16.9 g
Protein 4.4 g

445. Cheesecake Bites

Preparation Time: 20 minutes
Cooking Time: 2 minutes
Servings: 12
Ingredients:
8 oz. cream cheese, softened
½ cup plus 2 tablespoons sugar, divided
4 tablespoons heavy cream, divided
½ teaspoon vanilla extract
½ cup almond flour
Directions:
Beat the cream cheese, ½ cup of sugar, 2 tablespoons of heavy cream, and vanilla extract in a stand mixer bowl.
With a scooper, scoop the mixture onto a parchment paper-lined baking pan.
Freeze for about 30 minutes or until firm.
In a small bowl, place the remaining cream.
In another small bowl, add the almond flour and the remaining sugar and mix well.
Dip each cheesecake bite in cream and then coat with the flour mixture.
Air Fry within 2 minutes at 300 degrees F.
Arrange the pan in "Air Fry Basket" and insert it in the oven.
Serve warm.
Nutrition:
Calories 149
Fat 10.7 g
Cholesterol 28 mg
Sodium 60 mg
Carbs 11.7 g
Fiber 0.5 g
Sugar 10.1 g
Protein 2.5 g

446. Chocolate Bites

Preparation Time: 15 minutes
Cooking Time: 13 minutes
Servings: 8
Ingredients:
2 cups plain flour
2 tablespoons cocoa powder
½ cup icing sugar
Pinch of ground cinnamon
1 teaspoon vanilla extract
¾ cup chilled butter
¼ cup chocolate, chopped into 8 chunks
Directions:
Mix the flour, icing sugar, cocoa powder, cinnamon, and vanilla extract in a bowl.
Cut the butter and mix till a smooth dough form.
Divide the dough into 8 equal-sized balls.
Press 1 chocolate chunk in the center of each ball and cover it with the dough thoroughly.
Place the balls into the baking pan.
Set the cooking time to 8 minutes at 355 degrees F Air Fry.
After 8 minutes of cooking, set the temperature at 320 degrees F for 5 minutes.
Place the baking pan onto the wire rack to cool completely before serving.
Nutrition:
Calories 328
Fat 19.3 g
Cholesterol 47 mg
Sodium 128 mg
Carbs 35.3 g
Fiber 1.4 g
Sugar 10.2 g
Protein 4.1 g

447. Shortbread Fingers

Preparation Time: 15 minutes
Cooking Time: 12 minutes
Servings: 10
Ingredients:
1/3 cup caster sugar
1 2/3 cups plain flour
¾ cup butter
Directions:
Mix the sugar plus flour in a large bowl. Add the butter and mix until a smooth dough form.
Cut the dough into 10 equal-sized fingers. With a fork, lightly prick the fingers.
Place the fingers into the lightly greased baking pan.
Set the cooking time to 12 minutes on Air Fry at 355 degrees F.
Place the baking pan onto a wire rack to cool for about 5-10 minutes.
Now, invert the shortbread fingers onto a wire rack to completely cool before serving.
Nutrition:
Calories 223
Fat 14 g
Cholesterol 37 mg
Sodium 99 mg
Carbs 22.6 g
Fiber 0.6 g
Sugar 0.7 g
Protein 2.3 g

448. Berry Tacos

Preparation Time: 15 minutes
Cooking Time: 5 minutes
Servings: 2
Ingredients:
2 soft shell tortillas
4 tablespoons strawberry jelly
¼ cup fresh blueberries
¼ cup fresh raspberries
2 tablespoons powdered sugar
Directions:
Spread 2 tablespoons of strawberry jelly over each tortilla
Top each with berries evenly and sprinkle with powdered sugar.
Select "Air Fry," the cooking time to 5 minutes at 300 degrees F.
Arrange the tortillas in "Air Fry Basket" and insert it in the oven. Serve warm.
Nutrition:
Calories 216
Fat 0.8 g
Cholesterol 0mg
Sodium 11 mg
Carbs 53.2 g
Fiber 3 g
Sugar 38.7 g

Protein 1.7 g

449. Apple Pastries

Preparation Time: 15 minutes
Cooking Time: 10 minutes
Servings: 6

Ingredients:

½ of a large apple, peeled, cored, and chopped
1 teaspoon fresh orange zest, grated finely
½ tablespoon white sugar
½ teaspoon ground cinnamon
7.05 oz. prepared frozen puff pastry

Directions:

In a bowl, mix all items except puff pastry. Cut the pastry into 16 squares.
Place about a teaspoon of the apple mixture in the center of each square.
Fold each square into a triangle and press the edges slightly with wet fingers.
Then with a fork, press the edges firmly.
Select Air Fry, set the cooking time to 10 minutes at 390 degrees F.
Arrange the apple pastries in a greased "Air Fry Basket" and put it in the oven. Serve warm.

Nutrition:

Calories 198
Fat 12.7 g
Cholesterol 0 mg
Sodium 83 mg
Carbs 18.8 g
Fiber 1.1 g
Sugar 3.2 g
Protein 2.5 g

450. Marshmallow Pastries

Preparation Time: 10 minutes
Cooking Time: 5 minutes
Servings: 4

Ingredients:

4 phyllo pastry sheets, thawed
2 oz. butter, melted
¼ cup chunky peanut butter
4 teaspoons marshmallow fluff
Pinch of salt

Directions:

Brush 1 sheet of phyllo with butter.
Put a second sheet over the first one and brush it with butter.
Repeat until all 4 sheets are used.
Cut the phyllo layers in 4 (3x12-inch) strips.
Put 1 tablespoon of peanut butter and 1 teaspoon of marshmallow fluff on the underside of a strip of phyllo.
Carefully fold the tip of the sheet over the filling to make a triangle.
Fold it repeatedly in a zigzag until the filling is fully covered.
Air Fry to 5 minutes at 360 degrees F.
Arrange the marshmallow pastries in a greased "Air Fry Basket" and put it inside the air fryer oven.
Put a pinch of salt and serve warm.

Nutrition:

Calories 248
Fat 20.5 g
Cholesterol 30 mg
Sodium 268 mg
Carbs 12.7 g
Fiber 1.3 g
Sugar 2.6 g
Protein 5.2 g

451. Nutella Banana Pastries

Preparation Time: 15 minutes
Cooking Time: 12 minutes
Servings: 4

Ingredients:

1 puff pastry sheet
½ cup Nutella
2 bananas, peeled and sliced

Directions:

Cut the pastry sheet into 4 equal-sized squares.
Spread the Nutella on each square of pastry evenly.
Divide the banana slices over Nutella.
Fold each square into a triangle and with wet fingers, slightly press the edges.
Then with a fork, press the edges firmly.
Select Air Fry, then the cooking time to 12 minutes at 375 degrees F.
Arrange the pastries in a greased "Air Fry Basket" and insert it in the oven.
Serve warm.

Nutrition:

Calories 221
Fat 10 g
Cholesterol 26 mg
Sodium 103 mg
Carbs 31.6 g
Fiber 2.6 g
Sugar 14.4 g
Protein 3.4 g

452. Lemon Mousse

Preparation Time: 15 minutes
Cooking Time: 12 minutes
Servings: 2

Ingredients:

4 oz. cream cheese softened
½ cup heavy cream
2 tablespoon fresh lemon juice
4-6 drops liquid stevia
2 pinches salt

Directions:

Mix all the items listed in a bowl.
Transfer the mixture into 2 ramekins.
Press the "Power Button" of Air Fry Oven and turn the dial to select the "Air Bake" mode.
Press the Time button and again turn the dial to set the cooking time to 12 minutes.
Now push the Temp button and rotate the dial to set the temperature at 350 degrees F.
Press the "Start/Pause" button to start.
When the unit beeps to show that it is preheated, open the lid.
Arrange the ramekins over the "Wire Rack" and insert it in the oven.
Place the ramekins onto a wire rack to cool.
Refrigerate for at least 3 hours before serving.

Nutrition:

Calories 305
Fat 31 g
Cholesterol 103 mg
Sodium 337 mg
Carbs 2.7 g
Fiber 0.1 g
Sugar 0.5 g
Protein 5 g

453. Chocolate Pudding

Preparation Time: 20 minutes
Cooking Time: 12 minutes
Servings: 4

Ingredients:

½ cup butter
2/3 cup dark chocolate, chopped
¼ cup caster sugar
2 medium eggs
2 teaspoons fresh orange rind, finely grated
¼ cup fresh orange juice
2 tablespoons self-rising flour

Directions:

Microwave the butter and chocolate on high heat for about 2 minutes or until melted completely, stirring after every 30 seconds.
Remove from the microwave and stir the mixture until smooth.
Add the sugar and eggs and whisk until frothy.
Add the orange rind and juice, followed by flour and mix until well combined.
Divide mixture into 4 greased ramekins about ¾ full.
Set within 12 minutes at 355 degrees F.
Arrange the ramekins in "Air Fry Basket" and insert it in the oven.
Place the ramekins set aside to cool completely before serving.

Nutrition:

Calories 454
Fat 33.6 g
Cholesterol 149 mg
Sodium 217 mg
Total Carbs 34.2 g
Fiber 1.2 g
Sugar 28.4g
Protein 5.7 g

454. Vanilla Soufflé

Preparation Time: 15 minutes
Cooking Time: 23 minutes
Servings: 6

Ingredients:

¼ cup butter softened
¼ cup all-purpose flour
½ cup plus 2 tablespoons sugar, divided
1 cup milk
3 teaspoons vanilla extract, divided
4 egg yolks
5 egg whites
1 teaspoon cream of tartar
2 tablespoons powdered sugar

Directions:

In a bowl, add the butter and flour and mix until a smooth paste form.
In a medium pan, mix ½ cup of sugar and milk over medium-low heat and cook for about 3 minutes or until the sugar is dissolved, stirring continuously.
Add the flour mixture, whisking continuously, and simmer for about 3-4 minutes or until the mixture becomes thick.
Remove, then stir in 1 teaspoon of vanilla extract.
Set aside for about 10 minutes to cool.
In a bowl, add the egg yolks and 1 teaspoon of vanilla extract and mix well.
Add the egg yolk mixture into milk mixture and mix until well combined.
In another bowl, add the egg whites, cream of tartar, remaining sugar, and vanilla extract and with a wire whisk, beat until stiff peaks form.
Fold the egg white's mixture into the milk mixture.
Grease 6 ramekins and sprinkle each with a pinch of sugar.
Place mixture into the prepared ramekins, and with the back of a spoon, smooth the top surface.
Air Fry function, then set the cooking time to 16 minutes at 330 degrees F.
Place the ramekins onto a wire rack to cool slightly.
Dust it using the powdered sugar and serve warm.

Nutrition:

Calories 250
Fat 11.6 g
Cholesterol 163 mg
Sodium 107 mg
Carbs 29.8 g
Fiber 0.1 g
Sugar 25 g
Protein 6.8 g

455. Fudge Brownies

Preparation Time: 15 minutes
Cooking Time: 20 minutes
Servings: 8

Ingredients:

1 cup of sugar
½ cup butter, melted
½ cup flour
1/3 cup cocoa powder
1 teaspoon baking powder
2 eggs
1 teaspoon vanilla extract

Directions:

Grease a baking pan.
Whisk the sugar and butter in a large bowl.
Add the remaining ingredients and mix until well combined.
Place mixture into the prepared pan, and with the spatula's back, smooth the top surface.
Choose Air Fry, then set the cooking time to 20 minutes at 350 degrees F.
Arrange the pan in "Air Fry Basket" and insert it in the oven.
Place the baking pan onto a wire rack to cool completely.
Cut into 8 equal-sized squares and serve.

Nutrition:

Calories 250
Fat 13.2 g
Cholesterol 71 mg

Sodium 99 mg
Total Carbs 33.4 g
Fiber 1.3 g
Sugar 25.2 g
Protein 3 g

456. Walnut Brownies

Preparation Time: 15 minutes
Cooking Time: 22 minutes
Servings: 4

Ingredients:

½ cup chocolate, roughly chopped
1/3 cup butter
5 tablespoons sugar
1 egg, beaten
1 teaspoon vanilla extract
Pinch of salt
5 tablespoons self-rising flour
¼ cup walnuts, chopped

Directions:

Microwave the chocolate and butter on a high heat within 2 minutes, stirring after every 30 seconds. Remove from microwave and set aside to cool.
In another bowl, add the sugar, egg, vanilla extract, salt, and whisk until creamy and light.
Add the chocolate mixture and whisk until well combined.
Put the flour and walnuts and mix until well combined.
Line a baking pan with a greased parchment paper.
Place mixture evenly into the prepared baking pan and, with the back of the spatula.
Set the cooking time to 20 minutes at 355 degrees F.
Place the baking pan onto a wire rack to cool completely.
Cut into 4 equal-sized squares and serve.

Nutrition:

Calories 407
Fat 27.4g
Cholesterol 86 mg
Sodium 180 mg
Carbs 35.9 g
Fiber 1.5 g
Sugar 26.2 g
Protein 6 g

457. Air Fryer Oreos

Preparation time: 15 minutes
Cooking time: 8 minutes
Servings: 6

Ingredients:

1/2 cup total pancake mixture
1/3 cup water
cooking spray
9 chocolate Oreo cookies
1 tbsp confectioners' sugar or to flavor

Directions:

Mix pancake mix plus water until well blended.
Line an air fryer basket using parchment paper.
Spray parchment paper with non-stick cooking spray.
Dip each cookie to the pancake mix and put it in the jar. Be sure they're not touching; cook in batches if needed.
Preheat the air fryer to 400 degrees F. Insert basket and cook 4 to 5 minutes; reverse and cook till golden brown, 2-3 minutes longer. Sprinkle with confectioners' sugar.

Nutrition:

Calories: 160
Carbs: 25g
Fat: 7g
Protein: 1g

458. Air Fryer Churros

Preparation time: 15 minutes
Cooking time: 5 minutes
Servings: 4

Ingredients:

1/4 cup butter
1/2 cup milk
1 pinch salt
1/2 cup flour
2 eggs
1/4 cup white sugar
1/2 teaspoon ground cinnamon

Directions:

Melt butter in a saucepan over medium-high water.
Pour milk and then add salt.
Reduce heat to mild and carry to a boil, still stirring with a wooden spoon. Instantly add flour all at one time. Keep mixing until the dough comes together.
Remove from heat and let cool for 5 to 7 minutes. Mix in eggs with the wooden spoon till choux pastry comes together.
Spoon dough to a pastry bag fitted with a large star tip—pipe dough into pieces directly into the air fryer bowl.
Air fry churros in 340 degrees F (175 degrees C) for 5 minutes.
Meanwhile, blend sugar and cinnamon in a small bowl and then pour on a shallow plate.
Eliminate fried churros from the air fryer and roll from the cinnamon-sugar mix.

Nutrition:

Calories: 173
Carbs: 33g
Fat: 2g
Protein: 5g

459. Air Fryer Apple Fritters

Preparation time: 15 minutes
Cooking time: 10 minutes
Servings: 6

Ingredients:

cooking mist
1 cup whole-wheat flour
1/4 cup white sugar
1/4 cup milk
1 plant
1 1/2 tsp baking powder
1 pinch salt
2 tbsp white sugar
1/2 teaspoon ground cinnamon
1 apple peeled, cored, and sliced
Glaze:
1/2 cup confectioners' sugar
1 tbsp milk

1/2 tsp caramel infusion
1/4 teaspoon ground cinnamon

Directions:

Warm an air fryer to 350 degrees F (175 degrees C). Place a parchment paper down to the edge of the air fryer. Water with non-stick cooking spray.

Mix flour, 1/4 cup sugar, egg, butter, baking powder, and salt in a small pot. Stir once combined.

Mix 2 tbsp sugar cinnamon in another bowl and scatter over apples until coated. Mix apples to the flour mixture when combined.

Dip fritters with a cookie scoop in the middle of the air fryer bowl.

Air-fry 5 minutes in the preheated fryer. Flip fritters and cook until crispy, about 5 minutes longer.

Meanwhile, mix confectioners' sugar, butter, caramel extract, and cinnamon in a cup. Move fritters into a cooling system and drizzle with glaze.

Nutrition:

Calories: 300
Carbs: 26g
Fat: 20g
Protein: 5g

460. Air Fryer Roasted Bananas

Preparation time: 15 minutes
Cooking time: 8 minutes
Servings: 1

Ingredients:

1 banana, sliced diagonals
avocado oil cooking spray

Directions:

Line the air fryer basket using a parchment paper.

Warm an air fryer to 375 degrees F (190 degrees C).

Put banana pieces in the jar, making sure they are not touching; cook in batches if needed—mist banana pieces with avocado oil.

Cook at the air fryer for 5 minutes. Eliminate basket and reverse banana pieces carefully.

Cook till banana pieces are browning and caramelized, an extra 2-3 minutes. Carefully remove from the basket.

Nutrition:

Calories: 35
Carbs: 9g
Fat: 0g
Protein: 0g

461. Air Fryer Beignets

Preparation time: 15 minutes
Cooking time: 14 minutes
Servings: 4

Ingredients:

Cooking spray
1/2 cup all-purpose flour
1/4 cup white sugar
1/8 cup water
1 large egg, separated
1 1/2 tsp peanut butter
1/2 tsp baking powder
1/2 tsp vanilla extract
1 pinch salt
2 tbsp confectioners' sugar or to flavor

Directions:

Warm the air fryer to 370 degrees F (185 degrees C). Oil a silicone egg-bite meld with non-stick cooking spray.

Whisk rice, tea, sugar, egg yolk, butter, baking powder, vanilla extract, and salt in a large pot. Stir to mix.

Beat egg in a small bowl with an electric hand mixer on medium speed until soft peaks form. Fold into batter. Apply batter into the prepared mold with a tiny hinged ice cream spade.

Put lined silicone mold to the bucket of their air fryer. Fry from the preheated air fryer for about 10 minutes. Eliminate mold from the bottle; soda beignets out and turn over on a parchment paper across.

Place parchment around with beignets back in the air fryer bowl. Cook for another 4 minutes. Eliminate beignets in the air fryer bowl and sprinkle with confectioners ' sugar.

Nutrition:

Calories: 287
Carbs: 43g
Fat: 10g
Protein: 6g

462. Air-Fried Banana Cake

Preparation time: 15 minutes
Cooking time: 30 minutes
Servings: 3

Ingredients:

Cooking spray
1/3 cup brown sugar
3 1/2 tsp butter, at room temperature
1 banana, mashed
1 egg
2 tbsp honey
1 cup self-rising flour
1/2 teaspoon ground cinnamon
1 pinch salt

Directions:

Warm an air fryer to 320 degrees F (160 degrees C). Spray a tiny skillet pan with cooking spray.

Beat butter and sugar in a cup with an electric mixer until smooth. Blend potato, mango, and honey in another bowl. Whisk banana mix to butter mixture until smooth.

Sift the rice, cinnamon, and salt to the shared banana-butter mixture. Mix batter until dry, then shift to the prepared pan; degree the surface using the back of a spoon.

Put the cake pan from the air fryer bowl. Slide the basket to the air fryer and set the timer for thirty minutes. Serve.

Nutrition:

Calories: 135
Carbs: 23g
Fat: 4g
Protein: 1g

463. Air-Fried Butter Cake

Preparation time: 15 minutes
Cooking time: 15 minutes
Servings: 4

Ingredients:

cooking spray
7 tablespoons butter, at room temperature
1/4 cup white sugar
2 tbsp white sugar
1 egg
1 2/3 cups all-purpose flour
1 pinch salt, or to flavor
6 tsp milk

Directions:

Warm an air fryer to 350 degrees F (180 degrees C). Spray a tiny skillet pan with cooking spray.

Beat butter and 1/4 cup and 2 tbsp oil in a bowl with an electric mixer till smooth and white. Stir in the egg and mix until smooth and fluffy. Cover with salt and flour.

Remove milk and mix batter full. Turn batter into the prepared pan; use a spoon's back to weigh surface area.

Put the basket pan out of the air fryer. Set the timer for 15 minutes. Bake until a toothpick comes out clean, inserted into the cake.

Take the cake out of the pan and allow it to cool for around 5 minutes.

Nutrition:

Calories: 230
Carbs: 29g
Fat: 11g
Protein: 2g

464. Gluten-Free Fresh Cherry Crumble

Preparation time: 15 minutes
Cooking time: 25 minutes
Servings: 5

Ingredients:

One-third cup Butter
4 cups with black cherries
10 Tsp white sugar, split
2 Tsp orange juice
1 Top fermented pure cooked flour for use
1 Tsp Ground Vanilla
1 Tsp of field musk
1 clove of ground cinnamon

Directions:

Crush the butter and placed in the freezer for about 15 minutes, until solid.

Preheat air fryer to 325 ° F (165 ° C).

Blend in a bowl of pitted cherries, 2 tbsp of sugar, and lemon juice; mix well. Pour combination of cherry over the baking pot.

In a pot, whisk in flour and 6 tbsp of sugar. Split in fingered butter until the flakes are pea-sized.

Distribute the cherries over and softly push down.

In a cup, stir 2 tbsp of butter, vanilla paste, nutmeg, and cinnamon. Powder the sugar over the crust and the cherries.

Fry in the air fryer, preheated. Test at 25 minutes; or even browned, continue to test and cook for 5-minute intervals until slightly brown.

Open the door, and the air fryer turns off. Allow indoors to collapse for 10 minutes. Remove and allow to cool slowly, 5 minutes or so.

Nutrition:

Calories: 296
Carbs: 45g
Fat: 12g
Protein: 0g

465. Lime pudding

Preparation time: 15 minutes
Cooking time: 10 minutes
Servings: 4

Ingredients:

2 cups pulp lime
2 tbsp. zest lime
2 tops of milk
2 tbsp. powdered custard
3 tbsp. powdered sugar
3 tbsp. unsalted butter

Directions:

Boil the milk plus sugar in a saucepan, add the custard powder followed by the pear pulp, and then stir until a thick mixture is obtained.

Five minutes to preheat the fryer to 300 F. Put the dish and lower to 250 F, cook within 10 minutes.

Cool and serve.

Nutrition:

Calories: 110
Carbs: 18g
Fat: 3g
Protein: 2g

466. Mulberry Puddings

Preparation time: 15 minutes
Cooking time: 10 minutes
Servings: 6

Ingredients:

2 cups almond flour
1 cup of milk
2 tbsp. powdered custard
3 tbsp. powdered sugar
1 cup of mulberries juice
3 tbsp. unseasoned butter

Directions:

Boil the milk plus sugar, then add the custard powder followed by the almond flour and mulberry juice in a saucepan, then whisk until the mixture is thick.

Five minutes to preheat the fryer to 300 F. Adjust to 250 F, then cook within 10 minutes. Serve.

Nutrition:

Calories: 91
Carbs: 21g
Fat: 1g
Protein: 3g

467. Cauliflower Pudding

Preparation time: 15 minutes
Cooking time: 10 minutes
Servings: 6

Ingredients:

1 cup of flowering cauliflower
2 tops of milk
2 tbsp. powdered custard
3 tbsp. powdered sugar
3 tbsp. unseasoned butter

Directions:

Parboil the flowering cauliflower and placed on a plate.

Boil the milk plus sugar, then put the custard powder in a saucepan, and then whisk until the mixture is thick. Pour the mix over the florets.
Five minutes to warm the fryer to 300 F. Place the dish in the air fryer basket and adjust to 250 F. Cook within 10 minutes, then cool and serve.
Nutrition:
Calories: 120
Carbs: 11g
Fat: 8g
Protein: 3g

468. Peppermint Lava Cake

Preparation Time: 15 minutes
Cooking Time: 15 minutes
Servings: 4
Ingredients:
2 large eggs
2/3 cups semisweet chocolate chips
1 tsp. peppermint extract
½ cup cubed butter
6 tablespoons all-purpose flour
2 large egg yolks
2 tablespoons crushed peppermint candies (optional)
1 cup confectioners' sugar
Directions:
Preheat air fryer oven to 375F.
Dissolve the butter and chocolate chips in a safe microwave bowl for 30 seconds and stir until smooth.
Whisk in eggs, egg yolks, confectioners' sugars and extract until blended. Fold in flout
Grease and flour ramekins, pour batter into ramekins but avoid overfilling it
Place ramekins in the air fryer oven basket and cook for 10 to 15 minutes until a thermometer reads 160F.
Remove, then allow it to sit for 5 minutes, sprinkle with crush candies and enjoy.
Nutrition:
Calories 367
Fat 19.2 g
Carbs 53.6 g
Fiber 2.7 g
Sugar 37.8 g
Protein 6.4 g

469. Molten Lava Cake

Preparation Time: 10 minutes
Cooking Time: 10 minutes
Servings: 4
Ingredients:
1.5 tbsp self-rising flour
3.5 tbsp baker's sugar
3.5 oz unsalted butter
3.5 oz dark chocolate, chopped
2 eggs
Directions:
Preheat Your Air fryer oven to 375F, Grease, and flour 4 standard oven-safe ramekins.
Dissolve the dark chocolate plus butter in a safe microwave bowl for 3 minutes, stirring throughout.
Whisk the eggs plus sugar until pale.
Put the melted chocolate mixture into the egg mixture. Stir in flour and combine
Fill up the ramekins about 3/4 full with mixture and bake in a preheated air fryer oven at 375F for 10 minutes.
Remove and allow cool in a ramekin for 2 minutes.
Enjoy with a raspberry drizzle.
Nutrition:
Calories 70
Fat 0.2 g
Carbs 18 g
Fiber 1.6 g
Sugar 11.2 g
Protein 0.6 g

470. Zucchini Fritters

Preparation Time: 15 minutes
Cooking Time: 15 minutes
Servings: 8
Ingredients:
100 g Plain Flour
1 Medium Egg beaten
5 Tbsp Milk
150 g Grated Courgette
75 g Spring Onion thinly sliced
25 g Cheddar Cheese grated
1 Tbsp Mixed Herbs
Salt & Pepper
Directions:
Preheat the air fryer oven to 360F.
Grate the zucchini making sure to remove excess moisture.
Put plain flour into a bowl and add the seasoning.
Whisk the egg and milk and then add to the flour to make a smooth batter. Stir in the cheese, add in the zucchini and the spring onion, and mix well.
Make them into small burger shapes and place them in the air fryer oven.
Cook at a 360f temperature for 6 minutes or until fully cooked.
Serve with a dollop of mayonnaise.
Nutrition:
Calories 191
Fat 16.5
Carbs 14.8 g
Fiber 3.2 g
Sugar 9.7 g
Protein 6.8 g

471. Two Ingredients Air Fryer Oven Croutons

Preparation Time: 10 minutes
Cooking Time: 12 minutes
Servings: 2
Ingredients:
2 Slices Whole meal Bread
1 Tbsp Olive Oil
Directions:
Chop slices of bread into medium chunks and place in Air fryer oven.
Add olive oil and cook for 8 minutes on a 200c heat.
Serve over soup.
Nutrition:
Calories 369
Fat 31 g
Carbs 20 g

Fiber 0.1 g
Sugar 17.7 g
Protein 5.1 g

472. Strawberry Cupcakes

Preparation Time: 10 minutes
Cooking Time: 13 minutes
Servings: 4
Ingredients:
100 g Butter
100 g Caster Sugar
2 Medium Eggs
100 g Self Raising Flour
½ Tsp Vanilla Essence
50 g Butter
100 g Icing Sugar
½ Tsp Pink Food Coloring
1 Tbsp Whipped Cream
¼ Cup Fresh Strawberries blended
Directions:
Preheat air fryer oven to 170c.
Mix the butter plus sugar in a large mixing bowl until light and fluffy; add vanilla essence and beat in eggs one at a time (adding little flour after each egg). Then fold in the remaining flour.
Place them in little bun cases but don't fill the cases too much.
Place cupcakes in the air fryer oven and cook for 8 minutes at 170c.
Meanwhile, cream butter and gradually add icing sugar until you have a creamy mixture, then add food coloring, whipped cream, and blended strawberries and mix well.
Once the cupcakes are done, use a piping bag to add topping to them in circular motions.
Serve and enjoy
Nutrition:
Calories 317g
Fat 11.9 g
Carbs 14.8 g
Fiber 1.1 g
Sugar 8.3 g
Protein 5 g

473. Shortbread

Preparation Time: 10 minutes
Cooking Time: 28 minutes
Servings: 8
Ingredients:
Brownie:
250 g Self Raising Flour
175 g Butter
75 g Caster Sugar
30 g Cocoa Powder
Roses Chocolates
2 Tsp Vanilla Essence
Chocolate Chips
Directions:
Place flour, butter, and caster sugar in a bowl rub butter into the flour until it resembles breadcrumbs, then knead until you have a dough ball
Roll out dough with a rolling pin and cut into your favorite shapes using cookie cutters.
Use a grill pan or baking mat inside your air fryer oven to cook the dough.
Set to 360F, then cook for 10 minutes. Allow cooling before serving.
Nutrition:
Calories 271
Fat 15 g
Carbs 33 g
Fiber 1 g
Sugar 26 g
Protein 4 g

474. Mars Bar

Preparation Time: 10 minutes
Cooking Time: 40 minutes
Servings: 12
Ingredients:
225 g Self Raising Flour
100 g Butter
30 g Caster Sugar
6 Mars Bars
1 Tbsp Icing Sugar
Directions:
Place butter, caster sugar, and self-rising flour in a mixing bowl rub butter into the flour plus sugar until it resembles breadcrumbs.
Put the water to the breadcrumbs one bit at a time while mixing until it forms a dough and kneads until you have a soft pastry dough ball.
Roll out your pastry and cut into 6 similar sized pieces.
Roll each Mars bar up in each of the six strips until the mars bar is not visible.
Place your mars bars into the air fryer oven, spacing them.
Cook for 6 minutes at 360f. Sprinkle with icing sugar and serve.
Nutrition:
Calories 398
Fat 13.8 g
Carbs 33.6 g
Fiber 1 g
Sugar 9.3 g
Protein 1.8 g

475. Dark Chocolate Ganache

Preparation Time: 10 minutes
Cooking Time: 12 minutes
Servings: 6
Ingredients:
150 g Dark Chocolate
30 g Butter
4 Tbsp Greek Yoghurt
1 Tsp Honey
Directions:
Break up the dark chocolate into squares.
Place butter, honey, and dark chocolate into cake pan and place pan in an air fryer oven basket.
Cook for 2 minutes at320f. Stir and add in your Greek Yoghurt.
Nutrition:
Calories 253
Fat 8.9 g
Carbs 24.7 g

Fiber 1.2 g
Sugar 11.3 g
Protein 5.3 g

476. British Victoria Sponge

Preparation Time: 5 minutes
Cooking Time: 10 minutes
Servings: 3

Ingredients:

100 g Plain Flour
100 g Butter
100 g Caster Sugar
2 Medium Eggs
Cake Filling:
2 Tbsp Strawberry Jam
50 g Butter
100 g Icing Sugar
1 Tbsp Whipped Cream

Directions:

Preheat air fryer oven to 180c.
Grease a baking dish that can fit into Air fryer oven
Cream the butter and sugar until they are light and fluffy, beat in the eggs, add a little flour with each of them, and then gently fold in the flour's remainder.
Place the mixture into the tin and cook in the Air fryer oven for 15 minutes at 180C and then at 170C for 10 minutes.
Leave to cool and slice in the middle equally
Cream butter while gradually add the icing sugar and whipped cream until you have a thick and creamy mixture.
Add a layer of strawberry jam and then a layer of cake filling and then add your other sponge on top.
Enjoy!

Nutrition:

Calories 219
Fat 10g
Protein 3g
Carbs 0g
Sugar 5g

477. Yorkshire Pudding

Preparation Time: 5 minutes
Cooking Time: 45 minutes
Servings: 4

Ingredients:

1 Tbsp Extra Virgin Olive Oil
50 g Plain Flour
1 Small Egg
150 ml Whole Milk
Salt & Pepper

Directions:

Preheat your Air fryer oven to 240F.
Mix the plain flour plus the seasoning in a bowl, then put in the egg a little at a time while stirring gradually. Put the milk a little at a time until you have a mixture that is thick as the batter.
Place little olive oil in Pudding tins and place in the air fryer oven for 5 minutes or until smoking.
Pour your mixture half into the tin and place back in the Air fryer oven and cook at 200C for 15 minutes.

Nutrition:

Calories 581
Fat 23.8g
Protein 15.8g
Sugar 7g

478. Rutabaga Fries

Preparation Time: 5 minutes
Cooking Time: 14 minutes
Servings: 2

Ingredients:

1 kg Rutabaga
1 Tbsp Extra Virgin Olive Oil
2 Tsp Thyme
Salt & Pepper

Directions:

Peel rutabaga, then use a heavy-duty knife to slice your rutabaga into fries.
Place slices into a mixing bowl along with the rest of the ingredients and mix with your hands
Cook at 320F for 15 minutes. Shake and cook again for 5 minutes at 360F.
Serve with your favorite sauce.

Nutrition:

Calories 238
Fat 6g
Protein 1g
Sugar 4g

479. Soft Chocolate Brownies

Preparation Time: 5 minutes
Cooking Time: 14 minutes
Servings: 2

Ingredients:

2 tsp. vanilla essence
12g caster sugar
100g Self Raising flour
2 tablespoons water
2 medium eggs (beaten)
142ml milk
175g brown sugar
50g chocolate
125g butter

Directions:

Preheat air fryer oven to 180C.
Dissolve the butter plus chocolate in a bowl above pan over medium heat. Add brown sugar, medium egg, and vanilla essence then ad self-rising flour and mix properly
Pour mixture into a greased dish that can be contained in air fryer oven
Cook in air fryer oven at 180C for 15 minutes
While the brownie is cooking, mix caster sugar and water in a pan over medium heat until sugar is melted.
Turn up the heat and cook for 3 minutes until color turns light brown then take off and rest for 2 minutes
Add butter to sugar liquid until melted and slowly add the milk. Set aside to cool
When brownies are ready, chop into squares, place on the plate alongside sliced bananas, and cover with caramel sauce. Serve

Nutrition:

Calories 238
Fat 6g
Protein 1g
Carbs 0g

Sugar 4g

480. Chocolate Eclairs

Preparation Time: 5 minutes
Cooking Time: 35 minutes
Servings: 6
Ingredients:
Éclair dough
150ml water
50g butter
3 medium eggs
100g plain flour
Cream filling
1 tsp icing sugar
1 tsp. vanilla essence
150ml whipped cream
Chocolate topping
25g butter
1 tablespoon whipped cream
50g milk chocolate (chopped into chunks)
Directions:
Preheat air fryer oven to 180C.
Place fat in water and heat over medium heat.
Remove from heat and stir in flour then return to heat and stir until it forms a medium ball in the middle of the pan
Transfer to plate to cool then beat in eggs until mixture is smooth then make into éclair shapes
Place in air fryer oven and cook at 180C for 10 minutes then at 160C for 8 minutes
While the dough is cooking, mix vanilla essence with whipped cream and icing sugar until nice and thick
While eclairs are ready and cooling, make the chocolate topping by placing milk chocolate, butter, and whipped cream in a glass bowl. Put the bowl over a skillet of hot water, then mix well until chocolate melts
Cover éclairs with melted chocolate and serve
Nutrition:
Calories 471
Fat 24g
Protein 4.1g
Carbs 0g
Sugar 6g

481. Vanilla Souffle

Preparation Time: 5 minutes
Cooking Time: 5 minutes
Servings: 16
Ingredients:
¼ cup All-Purpose Flour
¼ cup Butter (softened)
1 cup Whole Milk
¼ cup Sugar
4 Egg Yolks
2 tsp Vanilla Extract
1 Vanilla Bean
5 Egg Whites
1 oz Sugar
1 tsp Cream of Tartar
Directions:
Mix the flour and butter to smooth paste.
Heat milk and dissolve the sugar in a pan and bring to a boil.
Add the flour and butter mixture to the boiling milk, whisk hard to ensure smoothness.
Simmer for several minutes until the mix thickens, then cool in an ice bath for 10 minutes
Take 6 3-ounce soufflé dishes, coat with butter and sugar (not mixed with the ingredients).
In another mixing bowl, quickly beat the egg yolks and vanilla extract and add to the cooling milk mixture.
Beat the egg whites, sugar, and cream of tartar until the egg whites form medium-stiff peaks.
Mix the egg whites into the soufflé base, then pour into the prepared baking dishes.
Preheat the Air fryer oven to 320°F, place 3 souffle dishes and cook for 12-15 minutes.
Serve with a sprinkle of powdered sugar.
Nutrition:
Calories 303
Fat 3g
Carbs 0g
Protein 0.5g
Sugar 4g

482.Lemon Curd Pavlova

Preparation time: 30 minutes
Cooking time: 60 minutes
Servings: 4
Ingredients:
Shell:
3 large egg whites
¼ teaspoon cream of tartar
¾ cup Swerve confectioners'-style sweetener
1 teaspoon grated lemon zest
1 teaspoon lemon extract
Lemon Curd:
1 cup Swerve confectioners'-style sweetener or powdered sweetener
½ cup lemon juice
4 large eggs
½ cup of coconut oil
For Garnish (Optional):
Blueberries
Swerve confectioners'-style sweetener
Directions:
Preheat the air fryer to 275°F. Thoroughly grease a 7-inch pie pan with butter or coconut oil.
Make the shell: In a small bowl, use a hand mixer to beat the egg whites and cream of tartar until soft peaks form. Slowly sprinkle in the sweetener and mix until it's completely incorporated.
Add the lemon zest and lemon extract and continue to beat with the hand mixer until stiff peaks form.
Spoon the mixture into the greased pie pan, then smooth it across the bottom, up the sides, and onto the rim to form a shell.
Cook within 1 hour, then turn off the air fryer and let the shell stand in the air fryer for 20 minutes.
While the shell bakes, make the lemon curd: In a medium-sized heavy-bottomed saucepan, whisk together the sweetener, lemon juice, and eggs.
Add the coconut oil and place the pan on the stovetop over medium heat. Once the oil is melted, constantly whisk until the mixture thickens and thickly coats the

back of a spoon, about 10 minutes. Do not allow the mixture to come to a boil.

Pour the lemon curd mixture through a fine-mesh strainer into a medium-sized bowl. Put the small bowl inside the bottom of a larger bowl filled with ice water and occasionally whisk until the curd is completely cold about 15 minutes.

Place the lemon curd over the shell and garnish with blueberries and powdered sweetener, if desired—store leftovers in the refrigerator for up to 4 days.

Nutrition:

Calories 332
Fat 33g
Protein 9g
Carbs 4g
Fiber 1g

483. Sweet Cream Cheese Wontons

Preparation time: 15 minutes
Cooking time: 5 minutes
Servings: 16

Ingredients:

1 egg mixed with a bit of water
Wonton wrappers
½ C. powdered erythritol
8 ounces softened cream cheese
Olive oil

Directions:

Mix sweetener and cream cheese together.

Layout the 4 wontons at a time, then cover with a dish towel to prevent drying out.

Place ½ of a teaspoon of cream cheese mixture into each wrapper. Dip finger into egg/water mixture and fold diagonally to form a triangle. Seal edges well.

Repeat with the remaining ingredients.

Place filled wontons into the Air fryer and cook 5 minutes at 400 degrees, shaking halfway through cooking.

Nutrition:

Calories: 303
Fat:3g
Protein:0.5g
Carbs: 0g
Sugar:4g

484. Apple Dutch Baby

Preparation time: 50 minutes
Cooking time: 16 minutes
Servings: 3

Ingredients:

For the Batter
2 large eggs
¼ cup all-purpose flour
¼ teaspoon baking powder
1½ teaspoons granulated sugar
Pinch kosher salt
½ cup whole milk
1 tablespoon butter, melted
½ teaspoon pure vanilla extract
¼ teaspoon ground nutmeg
For the Apples
2 tablespoon butter
4 tablespoons granulated sugar
¼ teaspoon ground cinnamon
¼ teaspoon ground nutmeg
1 small tart apple, peeled, cored, and sliced
Vanilla ice cream (optional), for serving

Directions:

Mix the eggs, flour, baking powder, sugar, and salt in a medium bowl. Whisk lightly, then slowly pour in the milk.

Whisk in the melted butter, vanilla, and nutmeg. Let the batter stand for 30 minutes.

For the apples: Place the butter in a 6 × 3-inch round heatproof pan, then place in the air fryer basket. Set the air fryer to 400°F for 2 minutes.

Mix 2 tablespoons of the sugar plus the cinnamon and nutmeg in a small bowl and stir until well combined.

When the pan is hot, and the butter is melted, brush some butter up the pan's sides. Sprinkle the spiced sugar mixture over the butter.

Arrange the apple slices in the pan in a single layer and sprinkle the remaining 2 tablespoons sugar over the apples.

Set again to 400°F to 2 minutes, or until the mixture bubbles.

Gently pour the batter over the apples. Set the air fryer to 350°F within 12 minutes, or until the pancake is golden brown around the edges, the center is cooked through, and a toothpick emerges clean. Serve immediately with ice cream, if desired.

Nutrition:

Calories: 281
Carbs: 46g
Fat: 8g
Protein: 7g

485. French Toast Bites

Preparation time: 5 minutes
Cooking time: 15 minutes
Servings: 8

Ingredients:

Almond milk
Cinnamon
Sweetener
3 eggs
4 pieces of wheat bread

Directions:

Preheat air fryer to 360 degrees. Whisk eggs and thin out with almond milk. Mix 1/3 cup of sweetener with lots of cinnamon.

Tear bread in half, ball up pieces, and press together to form a ball. Soak bread balls in egg and then roll into cinnamon sugar, making sure to coat thoroughly.

Place coated bread balls into the Air fryer and bake 15 minutes.

Nutrition:

Calories: 180
Carbs: 30g
Fat: 5g
Protein: 4g

486. Coconutty Lemon Bars

Preparation time: 5 minutes
Cooking time: 25 minutes
Servings: 12

Ingredients:

¼ cup cashew
¼ cup fresh lemon juice, freshly squeezed
¾ cup of coconut milk
¾ cup erythritol
1 cup desiccated coconut
1 teaspoon baking powder
2 eggs, beaten
2 tablespoons coconut oil
A dash of salt

Directions:

Preheat the air fryer for 5 minutes. In a mixing bowl, combine all ingredients. Use a hand mixer to mix everything. Put into a baking dish that will fit in the air fryer.

Bake for 25 minutes at 350°F or until a toothpick inserted in the middle comes out clean

Nutrition:

Calories: 180
Carbs: 26g
Fat: 8g
Protein: 2g

487. Bread Pudding with Cranberry

Preparation time: 15 minutes
Cooking time: 45 minutes
Servings: 4

Ingredients:

1-1/2 cups milk
2-1/2 eggs
1/2 cup cranberries1 teaspoon butter
1/4 cup & 2 tbsp white sugar
1/4 cup golden raisins
1/8 teaspoon ground cinnamon
3/4 cup heavy whipping cream
3/4 teaspoon lemon zest
3/4 teaspoon kosher salt
3/4 French baguettes, cut into 2-inch slices
3/8 vanilla bean, split and seeds scraped away

Directions:

Lightly grease baking pan of the air fryer with cooking spray. Spread baguette slices, cranberries, and raisins.

In a blender, blend well vanilla bean, cinnamon, salt, lemon zest, eggs, sugar, and cream. Pour over baguette slices. Let it soak for an hour—cover pan with foil.

For 35 minutes, cook at 330°F. Let it rest for 10 minutes. Serve and enjoy.

Nutrition:

Calories: 200
Carbs: 44g
Fat: 0g
Protein: 5g

488. Spiced Pears with Honey-Lemon Ricotta

Preparation time: 15 minutes
Cooking time: 8 minutes
Servings: 4

Ingredients:

2 large Bartlett pears
3 tablespoons butter, melted
3 tablespoons brown sugar
½ teaspoon ground ginger
¼ teaspoon ground cardamom
½ cup whole-milk ricotta cheese
1 tablespoon honey, plus additional for drizzling
1 teaspoon pure almond extract
1 teaspoon pure lemon extract

Directions:

Cut the pears on half lengthwise, then scoop out the core. Place the pear halves in a medium bowl, add the melted butter, and toss.

Add the brown sugar, ginger, and cardamom; toss to coat. Place the pear halves, cut side down, in the air fryer basket.

Set to 375°F for 8 to 10 minutes, or until the pears are lightly browned and tender, but not mushy.

Meanwhile, mix the ricotta, honey, and almond and lemon extracts in a medium bowl. Beat it using an electric mixer on medium speed until the mixture is light and fluffy, about 1 minute.

Divide the ricotta mixture among four small shallow bowls. Place a pear half, cut side up, on top of the cheese. Drizzle with additional honey and serve.

Nutrition:

Calories: 156
Carbs: 40g
Fat: 0g
Protein: 0g

489. Indian Toast & Milk

Preparation time: 15 minutes
Cooking time: 20 minutes
Servings: 4

Ingredients:

1 cup sweetened condensed milk
1 cup evaporated milk
1 cup half-and-half
1 teaspoon ground cardamom, plus additional for garnish
1 pinch saffron thread
4 slices white bread
2 to 3 tablespoons ghee or butter, softened
2 tablespoons crushed pistachios, for garnish (optional)

Directions:

In a 6 × 4-inch round heatproof pan, combine the condensed milk, evaporated milk, half-and-half, cardamom, and saffron. Stir until well combined.

Place the pan in the air fryer basket.

Set to 350°F for 15 minutes, stirring halfway through the cooking time. Remove the sweetened milk from the air fryer and set aside.

Cut each bread into two triangles, then brush each side with ghee. Put the bread in the air fryer basket.

Set the air fryer to 350°F for 5 minutes or until golden brown and toasty.

Remove the bread from the air fryer. Arrange two triangles in each of four wide, shallow bowls. Pour the hot milk mixture on top of the bread and let soak for 30 minutes.

Garnish with pistachios if using, and sprinkle with additional cardamom.

Nutrition:

Calories: 40
Carbs: 0g
Fat: 0g

Protein: 0g

490. Baked Apple

Preparation time: 15 minutes
Cooking time: 20 minutes
Servings: 25

Ingredients:

¼ C. water
¼ tsp nutmeg
¼ tsp. cinnamon
1 ½ tsp. melted ghee
2 tbsp. raisins
2 tbsp. chopped walnuts
1 medium apple

Directions:

Preheat your air fryer to 350 degrees.
Slice the apple in half and discard some of the flesh from the center.
Place into a frying pan. Mix remaining ingredients together except water. Spoon mixture to the middle of apple halves. Pour water overfilled apples.
Place pan with apple halves into the Air fryer, bake 20 minutes.

Nutrition:

Calories: 180
Carbs: 22g
Fat: 6g
Protein: 2g

491. Peanut Butter-Honey-Banana Toast

Preparation time: 15 minutes
Cooking time: 19 minutes
Servings: 6

Ingredients:

2 tablespoons butter, softened
4 slices white bread
4 tablespoons peanut butter
2 bananas, peeled and thinly sliced
4 tablespoons honey
1 teaspoon ground cinnamon

Directions:

Put the butter on one side of each slice of bread, then peanut butter on the other side.
Arrange the banana slices on top of each slice's peanut butter sides (about 9 slices per toast). Drizzle honey on top of the banana and sprinkle with cinnamon.
Cut each banana slice in half lengthwise so that it will better fit into the air fryer basket. Arrange two pieces of bread, butter sides down, in the air fryer basket. Set to 375°F for 5 minutes. Then again to 400°F for an additional 4 minutes, or until the bananas have started to brown. Repeat with remaining slices.

Nutrition:

Calories: 151
Carbs: 23g
Fat: 5g
Protein: 5g

492. Cinnamon Sugar Roasted Chickpeas

Preparation time: 15 minutes
Cooking time: 10 minutes
Servings: 2

Ingredients:

1 tbsp. sweetener
1 tbsp. cinnamon
1 C. chickpeas

Directions:

Preheat air fryer to 390 degrees. Rinse and drain chickpeas.
Mix all fixing and add to the air fryer. Cook 10 minutes.

Nutrition:

Calories: 131
Carbs: 20g
Fat: 4g
Protein: 4g

493. Grilled Peaches

Preparation Time: 10 minutes
Cooking time: 10 minutes
Servings: 2

Ingredients:

2 peaches, cut into wedges and remove pits
¼ cup butter, diced into pieces
¼ cup brown sugar
¼ cup graham cracker crumbs

Directions:

Arrange peach wedges on air fryer oven rack and air fry at 350 F for 5 minutes.
In a bowl, mix the butter, brown sugar, and graham cracker crumbs.
Turn peaches skin side down.
Spoon butter mixture over top of peaches and air fry for 5 minutes more.
Top with whipped cream and serve.

Nutrition:

Calories: 378
Fat: 24.4 g
Sodium: 0 mg
Carbs: 40.5 g
Fiber: 0 g
Sugar: 33.6 g
Protein: 2.3 g

494. Simple & Delicious Spiced Apples

Preparation Time: 10 minutes
Cooking time: 10 minutes
Servings: 4

Ingredients:

4 apples, sliced
1 tsp apple pie spice
2 tbsp. sugar
2 tbsp. ghee, melted

Directions:

Add apple slices into the mixing bowl. Add remaining ingredients on top of apple slices and toss until well coated.
Transfer apple slices to air fryer oven pan and air fry at 350 F for 10 minutes.
Top with ice cream and serve.

Nutrition:

Calories: 196
Total Fat: 6.8 g
Cholesterol: 16 mg
Sodium: 0 mg
Carbs: 37.1 g
Fiber: 0 g

Sugar: 29.2 g
Protein: 0.6 g

495. Delicious Brownies

Preparation Time: 10 minutes
Cooking time: 33 minutes
Servings: 6

Ingredients:

2 eggs
½ cup walnuts, chopped
¼ cup all-purpose flour
1 cup brown sugar
1 ½ tsp vanilla
¼ cup of cocoa powder
½ cup butter
Pinch of salt

Directions:

Spray air fryer shallow baking dish with cooking spray and set aside.
In a microwave-safe bowl, combine butter and cocoa powder and microwave until butter is melted. Stir to combine and set aside to cool.
Once the butter mixture is cool, then whisk in eggs and vanilla.
Stir in brown sugar, walnuts, flour, and salt.
Put the batter into the prepared baking dish and bake in an air fryer oven at 320 F for 33 minutes.
Allow to cool completely, then slice and serve.

Nutrition:

Calories: 343
Fat: 23.5 g
Cholesterol: 95 mg
Sodium: 0 mg
Carbs: 30.9 g
Fiber: 0 g
Sugar: 23.9 g
Protein: 5.7 g

496. Tangy Mango Slices

Preparation Time: 10 minutes
Cooking time: 12 hours
Servings: 6

Ingredients:

4 mangoes peel and cut into ¼-inch slices
1/4 cup fresh lemon juice
1 tbsp. honey

Directions:

Mix the lemon juice plus honey in a bowl and set aside.
Add mango slices in lemon-honey mixture and coat well.
Arrange mango slices on air fryer rack and dehydrate at 135 F for 12 hours.

Nutrition:

Calories: 147
Fat: 0.9 g
Cholesterol: 0 mg
Sodium: 0 mg
Total Carbs: 36.7 g
Fiber: 0 g
Sugar: 33.7 g
Protein: 1.9 g

497. Peanut Butter Cookies

Preparation Time: 10 minutes
Cooking time: 5 minutes
Servings: 24

Ingredients:

1 egg, lightly beaten
1 cup of sugar
1 cup creamy peanut butter

Directions:

Mix egg, sugar, and peanut butter in a mixing bowl until well combined.
Spray air fryer oven tray with cooking spray.
Using an ice cream scooper, scoop out cookie onto the tray and flattened them using a fork.
Bake cookie at 350 F for 5 minutes.
Cook remaining cookie batches using the same temperature.
Serve and enjoy.

Nutrition:

Calories: 97
Fat: 5.6 g
Cholesterol: 7 mg
Sodium: 0 mg
Carbs: 10.5 g
Fiber: 0 g
Sugar: 9.4 g
Protein: 2.9 g

498. Dried Raspberries

Preparation Time: 10 minutes
Cooking time: 15 hours
Servings: 4

Ingredients:

4 cups raspberries wash and dry
1/4 cup fresh lemon juice

Directions:

Add raspberries and lemon juice in a bowl and toss well.
Arrange raspberries on air fryer oven tray and dehydrate at 135 F for 12-15 hours.
Store in an air-tight container

Nutrition:

Calories: 68
Fat: 0.9 g
Cholesterol: 0 mg
Sodium: 0 mg
Carbs: 15 g
Fiber: 0 g
Protein: 1.6 g

499. Peanut Butter Banana Bites

Preparation Time: 5 minutes
Cooking time: 6 minutes
Servings: 6

Ingredients:

6 wonton wrappers
1/2 cup of peanut butter
2 teaspoons of vegetable oil
1 large banana, sliced

Directions:

Set Air fryer to 380 degrees F for 6 minutes. Arrange 1 teaspoon of peanut butter and 1 banana slice in the middle of each wonton wrapper.

Drench the wrapper edges with water and seal the opposite sides. Place the wrappers on the cooking tray and drizzle with oil.
Flip the sides when it displays "Turn Food." Remove, and serve warm.

Nutrition:

Calories: 253 Cal
Fat: 12.9 g
Sodium: 0 mg
Carbs: 27.9 g
Fiber: 0 g
Sugar: 0 g
Protein: 8.8 g

500. Healthy Apple Crisp

Preparation Time: 5 minutes
Cooking time: 20 minutes
Servings: 4

Ingredients:

1/3 cup of quick oats
1/4 cup of brown sugar
2 tablespoons of light butter melted
1/2 teaspoon of cinnamon
3 cups of apples chopped
1 tablespoon of pure maple syrup
2 teaspoons of lemon juice
3 tablespoons of almond flour

Directions:

Set to 350 degrees F for 20 minutes. Combine apples with lemon juice, 1 tablespoon almond flour, cinnamon, and maple syrup in a bowl.
Mingle oats, melted butter, brown sugar, and remaining almond flour in another bowl, then pour the oats mixture into the apple's mixture. Transfer this mixture on the cooking tray.
Insert the cooking tray in the air fryer oven, flip the sides when it displays "Turn Food." Serve warm.

Nutrition:

Calories: 213
Fat: 14 g
Carbs: 55 g
Fiber: 0 g
Sugar: 0 g
Protein: 12 g

CPSIA information can be obtained
at www.ICGtesting.com
Printed in the USA
BVHW061352081220
595179BV00007B/477

9 781801 241984